COOKING THE NEW
DIABETIC
—— WAY ——
THE HIGH FIBRE
CALORIE-CONSCIOUS COOKBOOK

BRITISH DIABETIC ASSOCIATION

Diabetes affects nearly two per cent of the UK population. Although it cannot be cured or prevented, it can be controlled by proper treatment.

The *British Diabetic Association* (BDA) was formed in 1934 to help all diabetics, to overcome prejudice and ignorance about diabetes, and to raise money for research towards a cure. The Association is currently budgeting £1 million each year to this end, and is the largest single contributor to diabetic research in the UK.

The BDA is an independent organization with over 100,000 members and more than 300 local groups throughout the UK. It provides practical advice and information for diabetics, their families and those who work with them.

Educational and activity holidays are organized for diabetics of all age groups, plus teach-in weekends for families with newly-diagnosed children or teenagers. The BDA also publishes a wide range of helpful books, leaflets, videos and goods.

Every two months, the BDA also publishes a magazine, 'Balance', which keeps readers up-to-date with news, views and comments about all aspects of diabetes and the latest research. 'Balance' is sent free to all members, or is available from newsagents price 85p.

All diabetics, whatever their treatment, follow a lifelong diet and 'Balance' publishes recipes and dietary information to help bring interest and variety in eating.

Membership of the BDA is open to anyone and new members are welcomed. The subscription rates are:

Annual Membership:	£5 per year
Pensioner Membership:	£1 per year
Reduced Rate Membership:	£1 per year
(widows on government grants/	
unemployed/disabled)	
Life Membership:	£105 single payment or
	7 years under covenant at £15 per year
	(forms available on request)

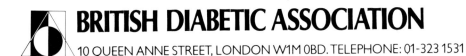

BRITISH DIABETIC ASSOCIATION
10 QUEEN ANNE STREET, LONDON W1M 0BD. TELEPHONE: 01-323 1531

COOKING THE NEW
DIABETIC
WAY
THE HIGH FIBRE
CALORIE-CONSCIOUS COOKBOOK

Compiled by Jill Metcalfe
Dietitian at The British Diabetic Association

With a foreword by Sir Harry Secombe CBE

WARD LOCK LIMITED · LONDON

ACKNOWLEDGEMENTS

The British Diabetic Association would like to thank Mrs Shirley Whitehouse of Tunbridge Wells for originating many of the recipes in this book.

Mrs Whitehouse, a diabetic on insulin, recognized the difficulties of controlling her own weight by a carbohydrate counted diet. She, therefore, utilized her experience as a health and cookery writer to produce a range of low fat recipes to help control her own calorie intake and thereby prevent a gain in weight.

Recognizing the value of these recipes, the BDA developed them and others into a selection of low fat/high fibre dishes which constitute the basis of this book.

Inside photography   Eric Carter
Home Economist for photography   Roz Denny
Home Economist for recipe development
    Joanne Murray

The BDA and publisher would also like to thank Harrods Ltd for kindly loaning equipment for photography.

First published in Great Britain in 1983
by Ward Lock Limited, 8 Clifford Street,
London W1X 1RB, an Egmont Company
Reprinted 1987

Text filmset in Helvetica
by A.K.M. Associates (U.K.) Ltd., Southall.

Printed and bound in Singapore by Toppan Printing Company Ltd.

British Library Cataloguing in Publication Data

Metcalfe, Jill
    Cooking the new diabetic way.
    1. Diabetes – Diet therapy – recipes
    I. Title
    641.5'6314   RC662

    ISBN 0-7063-6581-X

Contents

Foreword

As a diabetic, I realize too well the importance of following a diet. It was only when I became quite ill that I started to take my diet seriously. Since I have buckled down to it, I feel much better, am enjoying life and am looking forward to many more healthy years with my family.

I am delighted to be associated with this book which represents a new and fresh approach to diabetic cookery for weightwatchers.

Sir Harry Secombe CBE
PRESIDENT
The British Diabetic Association

The Aim of This Book

This book introduces a new and healthy approach in reduced calorie cooking. It is not, nevertheless, an exaltation of the lettuce leaf, but an array of new tastes and flavours created from basic everyday ingredients. The recipes will help and delight all diabetic slimmers and weightwatchers as well as anyone else who is trying to plan healthy and interesting low calorie meals.

In more detail, recent research has shown that there are two things which are essential to a satisfactory low calorie diet. It must be low in fat and high in fibre.

A low fat/high fibre diet is very beneficial to health in many ways, but it has special value to the slimmer. Fats are the most calorie-concentrated foods we eat, so the case for reducing them is self-evident. Fibre is of particular value to people on a low calorie diet because it makes for more satisfying and filling food without adding too many calories. Remember too, that a satisfying diet is an easier one to follow.

A high fibre diet is also of particular importance to diabetics as it helps them gain a better control of the condition.

Additionally, at least half those affected by diabetes are advised to lose weight as a way – often the only one needed – of stabilizing the condition. Many more need help with weight control at some stage in their life. In the past there has tended to be some confusion between the dietary advice diabetics have been given for controlling the condition, ie to eat less sugar and more fibre, and the advice they have been given to help them lose weight, ie to eat less calories by reducing fatty foods.

Cooking the New Diabetic Way sets out to clarify this situation by presenting recipes which, for the first time, combine the principles of both diabetic control and weight loss.

While many slimmers lose weight by revising their diets to include more fibre and less fat and sugar, many prefer the added discipline of either calorie or carbohydrate counting. This is also the first book to have calorie and carbohydrate counted, low fat/high fibre recipes.

Adapting Your Diet to Lose Weight

If you eat more calories than your body requires to meet the demands you make of it from day to day, then you become overweight. The first stage in losing weight by calorie control is, therefore, to establish what your calorie intake is at present and to plan a diet which provides substantially less.

Of limited value and often indeed harmful, are the charts, found in magazines, newspapers and books, which categorize people by sex, age, occupation and so on and then recommend a calorie intake for each group. Each individual has different demands, and it is essential to take the greatest care in estimating your own particular calorie intake when working out a diet appropriate to your needs.

The best approach to the problem – and one which is strongly recommended to diabetics – is to consult a dietitian who will estimate accurately your present calorie intake, and give guidance on appropriate calorie targets and well-balanced meals.

If you do not have access to a dietitian, you can estimate your own calorie intake in the following way:

Keep a detailed record for three days, including one typical weekend day, of everything you eat and drink. Then, using the Food Values chart on pages 142–46, calculate the approximate number of calories provided by each day's day's food and drink. (Figures for packaged foods are available from the British Diabetic Association in their booklet *Countdown*.) Add together the calorie intake for the three days, and divide the total by three. This figure represents your average daily calorie intake on your present diet.

To lose weight you will need to reduce this figure by about one-third. In some cases a bigger or smaller reduction will be required, but one-third is a useful and realistic initial reduction.

If you are a diabetic *not* on tablets or insulin, you should divide this reduced daily calorie intake evenly between your three main meals or, if you prefer, between your three main meals plus snacks.

If you are a diabetic on tablets or insulin and have been prescribed a carbohydrate allowance, you need to estimate your present carbohydrate intake as well as your calorie intake. If you find that you are keeping to your prescribed allowance, then your present carbohydrate intake and its distribution through the day should be maintained, but your present calorie intake should be reduced by one-third; this quantity should then be spread evenly through the day. If, on the other hand, you find that you are exceeding your prescribed carbohydrate allowance, your calorie intake should be reduced by one-third and about half those calories planned to be provided by carbohydrate. (The chart opposite will help here.) The distribution of your carbohydrate through the day should continue as originally prescribed. Once the new diet has been established, it is important to consult your doctor as he may need to adjust your medication with the likely improvement in your diabetic control.

Carbohydrate Content of the Diet
On 1000   calories a day, aim at 120 grams   carbohydrate (CHO)
On 1200   calories a day, aim at 150 grams   carbohydrate (CHO)
On 1500   calories a day, aim at 180 grams   carbohydrate (CHO)
On 1800   calories a day, aim at 220 grams   carbohydrate (CHO)
On 2000   calories a day, aim at 250 grams   carbohydrate (CHO)
On 2200   calories a day, aim at 270 grams   carbohydrate (CHO)

About the Recipes

1) Recipe ingredients are given in both imperial and metric measurements. You should follow one system or the other. Mixing the two will produce inferior results and will also make the calorie and carbohydrate calculations inaccurate.

2) All the recipes include a calculation of the total number of calories and the total amount of carbohydrate they contain. These have been rounded up to the nearest 10 calories and 5 grams carbohydrate. Where the carbohydrate total is less than 10 grams, this is stated on the recipe as negligible (neg). The calculations are based on the metric version of the recipe, so diabetics requiring complete accuracy should use the metric measurements.

   Diabetics are being urged to aim at providing half their energy (calories) from carbohydrate sources. Since vegetables in quantity make a significant contribution, the carbohydrate calculations include the available carbohydrate contributed by the vegetables in each recipe.

3) The recipes are for either two or four average servings. If you prefer or need to have a large or smaller portion of a particular recipe, divide the total carbohydrate and calorie figures by the number of servings obtained from that recipe.

   For example:
Mustard pork and mushrooms (page 43) has total CHO 60g, total calories 860.
   Divided into four equal servings, each portion contains
   15g CHO and 215 calories (60g CHO ÷ 4 = 15g CHO;
   860 cals ÷ 4 = 215 calories)

   Divided into six smaller servings, each portion contains
   10g CHO and approx 145 calories (60g CHO ÷ 6 = 10g CHO;
   860 cals ÷ 6 = 145 calories (approx))
   The importance of reducing the fat in your cooking to a minimum cannot be overstressed. Every gram of fat you avoid saves nine calories. Save just 10 grams and you have saved 90 calories. When you are trying to keep to 1200 calories a day, 90 calories saved is no mean achievement. So follow carefully any instruction in a recipe to trim meat or to drain off any excess fat or oil.

4) Weights given for ingredients are for the food before any preparation has taken place, unless otherwise stated, eg 50g/2 oz brown rice, cooked implies 50g/2 oz uncooked brown rice; but 50g/2 oz cooked brown rice implies exactly what is stated, ie 50g/2 oz cooked weight. For the convenience of the cook, vegetables are often listed in the ingredients by size rather than weight. It is assumed that a small onion weighs about 50g/2 oz, a medium onion, carrot or pepper weighs about 100g/4 oz, and a large onion, carrot or pepper weighs about 225g/8 oz. Where fresh fruit such as berries are indicated, the equivalent weight of frozen fruit can be substituted. Thaw and use as required.

5) Can or carton sizes are sometimes specified. Small variations from these standard sizes will not, however, make an appreciable difference to the success of the recipe or to the calculations.

6) Where herbs are used, these are dried, unless otherwise indicated.

7) A serving suggestion follows many recipes. In the case of main course dishes, this is designed to produce a well-balanced meal. If a recipe is quite high in calories, a low calorie accompaniment is suggested. Similarly, if a recipe is not very rich in fibre, the recommended accompaniment makes up for this. Where vegetables are indicated, they should be cooked plainly, without fat. Of course, you may prefer to substitute your own ideas to fit in with your individual calorie or carbohydrate plan.

Note   The calorie and carbohydrate values of the foods contained in the serving suggestions have not been included in the recipe calculations.

8) Basic kitchen equipment is all that is required to follow the recipes. This must include accurate scales, a measuring jug and a set of standard measuring spoons. Frying pans, saucepans and baking tins should be non-stick so that a minimum amount of fat or oil may be used in cooking. In addition, a dry-fry pan, in which you can fry anything without adding oil or fat, is an excellent piece of equipment; a blender (liquidizer) is very useful for making soups and purées, although it is essential for only a very few recipes; and a pressure cooker saves a lot of cooking time, particularly for dried peas, beans and lentils.

9) A well stocked store cupboard and refrigerator will help you keep to your diet. The following is a list of foods which it is useful always to have in stock:

Dry and packaged goods
Wholemeal or wholewheat flour, brown rice, wholewheat pasta, gelatine, a variety of dried fruit, dried peas, dried beans, lentils, stock cubes, Worcestershire sauce, cider or wine vinegar, lemon juice, sugar-free mixers and squashes, fructose (fruit sugar) liquid sweetener, dried herbs and spices

Canned foods
Mackerel and tuna in brine, frankfurters in brine, tomatoes, sweetcorn, broad beans, butter beans, red kidney beans, tomato juice, concentrated tomato purée, canned fruit without added sugar

Refrigerated and frozen foods
A variety of seafood such as plain fish fillets, shrimps and prawns, frozen vegetables, good quality stewing beef, stewing lamb and 'free-flow' mince, low fat spread, skimmed milk, natural yoghurt

Prepared foods
A small supply of cold brown rice or wholewheat pasta is very useful to serve with salads and other cold dishes. Cook in the normal way, with any seasoning, then pour plenty of boiling water over the cooked rice or pasta, and drain well. Cover securely, and leave in a refrigerator for up to a week

Soups and Starters

A well-chosen soup or starter can turn the most ordinary meal into an occasion. If you are slimming, the vegetables also provide a very pleasant way of taking the edge off your appetite so you finish your main course quite satisfied and can resist the temptation of reaching for an unsuitable dessert.

A great advantage of soups is that they can be prepared in quantity and frozen, or kept for several days in a refrigerator. Why not keep a variety of soups in this way to ring the changes on your everyday diet?

Soups

Aubergine Soup

1 large aubergine, skinned and chopped
1 large onion, finely chopped
2 medium tomatoes, deseeded and
  chopped
1 medium green pepper, deseeded and
  chopped
2 cloves garlic, crushed
1 × 5ml spoon/1 teaspoon basil

275ml/½ pint cold water
1 chicken stock cube
150g/5.3 oz natural yoghurt (1 small
  carton)
salt, pepper

Garnish
fresh mint, chopped

Put the aubergine, onion, tomatoes, pepper, garlic and basil into a large saucepan, add the water and crumble in the stock cube. Heat slowly to boiling point, reduce the heat, cover and simmer for 30 minutes. Remove from the heat, cool slightly, then stir in the yoghurt. Season to taste, and garnish with chopped mint.

Serves 2

Total CHO   **30g**
Total calories **180**

Celery and Fennel Soup

4 stalks celery, trimmed and chopped
½ head of fennel, trimmed and sliced
1 small onion, chopped
1 clove of garlic, crushed
salt, pepper

550ml/1 pint cold water
1 chicken stock cube

Garnish
paprika

Put the vegetables, garlic and seasoning into a large saucepan. Add the water and crumble in the stock cube. Heat to boiling point, reduce the heat, cover and simmer for 30 minutes. Season to taste, and garnish with paprika.

Serves 2

Total CHO   **neg**
Total calories **80**

Cream of Cauliflower Soup

1 small cauliflower, trimmed and
  chopped
550ml/1 pint cold water
1 chicken stock cube
1 × 15ml spoon/1 tablespoon skimmed
  milk

salt, pepper

Garnish
fresh parsley, chopped

Put the cauliflower into a saucepan with the water, and
crumble in the stock cube. Heat to boiling point, reduce the
heat, cover and simmer for 30 minutes. Add the skimmed
milk, season to taste, and garnish with parsley.

Serves 2

Total CHO   **neg**
Total calories   **60**

Green Bean Soup

225g/8 oz whole green beans
1 small head of celery, trimmed and
  chopped
275ml/½ pint tomato juice

275ml/½ pint cold water
1 chicken stock cube
a dash of soy sauce

Put the vegetables, tomato juice and water into a saucepan
and crumble in the stock cube. Heat to boiling point, reduce
the heat, cover and simmer for 30 minutes. Season to
taste and, just before serving, add a dash of soy sauce.

Serves 2

Total CHO   **10g**
Total calories   **120**

Lettuce Soup

1 lettuce, shredded
1 medium onion, chopped
3 × 15ml spoons/3 tablespoons
  skimmed milk
1 clove of garlic, crushed
salt, pepper

550ml/1 pint cold water
1 chicken stock cube

Garnish
1 × 15ml spoon/1 tablespoon natural
  yoghurt

Put the lettuce, onion, milk, garlic and seasoning in a
saucepan. Add the water and crumble in the stock cube. Heat
to boiling point, reduce the heat, cover and simmer for 30
minutes. Season to taste and stir the yoghurt into the soup to
garnish.

Serves 2

Total CHO   **neg**
Total calories   **60**

15

Chicken Soup

1 chicken leg
1 medium onion, chopped
2 large carrots, sliced
4 stalks celery, trimmed and chopped

salt, freshly ground black pepper
550ml/1 pint cold water
1 chicken stock cube

Put the chicken, vegetables and seasoning in a large saucepan. Add the water and crumble in the stock cube. Heat to boiling point, reduce the heat, cover and simmer for 1 hour. Cool slightly and remove the meat from the bone. Season to taste and sprinkle with freshly ground black pepper.

Serves 2

Total CHO   *10g*
Total calories *280*

Gazpacho de Españã

550ml/1 pint tomato juice
1 clove of garlic, crushed
5 × 10ml spoons/5 dessertspoons
  wine vinegar
a pinch of basil
celery salt
freshly ground black pepper

Accompaniments
1 size 3 egg, hard-boiled and chopped
1 medium green pepper, deseeded
  and chopped
1 stalk of celery, trimmed and finely
  chopped
½ small cucumber, peeled and cubed

Sieve the tomato juice, garlic and vinegar or process in a blender. Season to taste and chill in a refrigerator before serving.
   Put the egg, pepper, celery and cucumber in separate glass dishes and serve with the gazpacho.

Serves 2

Total CHO   *20g*
Total calories *200*

Tomato Consommé

550ml/1 pint tomato juice
1 small onion, chopped
2 bay leaves
a pinch of basil

celery salt
white pepper
2 beef stock cubes

Put the tomato juice, onion, herbs and seasoning into a saucepan and crumble in the stock cubes. Heat to boiling point, reduce the heat, cover and simmer for 30 minutes. Remove the bay leaves, season to taste, cool, and then sieve, or process in a blender. Serve cold, or re-heat and serve hot.

Serves 2

Total CHO   *20g*
Total calories *100*

Tomato Soup

2 large tomatoes, chopped
1 clove of garlic, crushed
150ml/¼ pint skimmed milk

1 × 15ml spoon/1 tablespoon fresh
  parsley, chopped
salt, pepper
1 chicken stock cube

Put the tomato, garlic, milk, parsley and seasoning in a
saucepan and crumble in the stock cube. Heat to boiling
point, reduce the heat, cover and simmer for 30 minutes.
Cool, then season to taste and sieve, or process in a blender.

Serves 2

Total CHO   ***neg***
Total calories   ***50***

Cabbage Soup

450g/1 lb white cabbage, shredded
1 medium onion, chopped
275ml/½ pint tomato juice
salt, pepper
275ml/½ pint cold water

1 beef stock cube

Garnish
fresh parsley, chopped

Put the cabbage, onion, tomato juice, seasoning and water in
a large saucepan, and crumble in the stock cube. Heat to
boiling point, reduce the heat, cover and simmer for 45
minutes. Season to taste, and garnish with chopped parsley.

Serves 4

Total CHO   ***20g***
Total calories   ***120***

Cream of Celery Soup

1 large head of celery, trimmed and
  chopped
1 medium red pepper, deseeded and
  chopped
25g/1 oz fresh chives, chopped

550ml/1 pint water
1 chicken stock cube
150ml/¼ pint skimmed milk
salt, pepper

Put the celery, pepper and chives into a saucepan, add the
water and crumble in the stock cube. Heat to boiling point,
reduce the heat, cover and simmer for 30 minutes. Sieve, or
process in a blender for 2 minutes. Return to the saucepan
and add the milk, then simmer for a further 10 minutes.
Season to taste.

Serves 4

Total CHO   ***10g***
Total calories   ***100***

Serving suggestion Wholemeal toast

Leek and Chick-pea Soup

100g/4 oz chick-peas
450g/1 lb leeks
3 × 15ml spoons/3 tablespoons
  Worcestershire sauce
3 × 15ml spoons/3 tablespoons
  concentrated tomato purée

salt, pepper
550ml/1 pint water
2 chicken stock cubes

Garnish
fresh parsley, chopped

Serves 4

Soak the chick-peas in water overnight. Put in a large
saucepan with the leeks, Worcestershire sauce, tomato pureé
and seasoning. Add the water, and crumble in the stock
cubes. Heat to boiling point, reduce the heat, cover and
simmer for 1½ hours or until the chick-peas are tender.
Alternatively, cook in a pressure cooker. Season to taste and
garnish with chopped parsley.

Total CHO   80g
Total calories   380

Country Soup

1 small onion, chopped
1 large leek, trimmed and sliced
225g/8 oz white cabbage, shredded
2 courgettes, finely sliced
2 large tomatoes, skinned and chopped
50g/2 oz brown rice
fresh parsley, chopped
1 × 2.5ml spoon/½ teaspoon basil
1 × 5ml spoon/1 teaspoon tarragon

3 whole cloves
2 cloves garlic, crushed
freshly ground black pepper
1 × 2.5ml spoon/½ teaspoon celery salt
1100ml/2 pints water
2 × 15ml spoons/2 tablespoons
  concentrated tomato pureé
1 beef stock cube

Serves 4

Put the vegetables, rice, herbs, cloves, garlic and seasoning
in a large saucepan. Add the water and tomato pureé, and
crumble in the stock cube. Heat to boiling point, reduce the
heat, cover and simmer for 45 minutes. Leave to stand for
24 hours, then remove the cloves, reheat thoroughly and
serve hot.

Total CHO   60g
Total calories   340

Winter Soup

1 large head of celery, trimmed and
  chopped
450g/1 lb leeks, trimmed and sliced
2 medium tomatoes, chopped
2 bay leaves

2 × 15ml spoons/2 tablespoons
  Worcestershire sauce
celery salt
freshly ground black pepper
550ml/1 pint cold water
2 beef stock cubes

Put the vegetables, herbs, Worcestershire sauce and
seasoning in a saucepan. Add the water and crumble in the
stock cubes. Heat to boiling point, reduce the heat, cover and
simmer for 45 minutes. Remove the bay leaves and season to
taste.

Serving suggestion Wholemeal toast

Serves 4

Total CHO   *20g*
Total calories *120*

Cream of Courgette Soup

450g/1 lb courgettes, sliced
1 medium onion, chopped
1 clove of garlic, crushed
sprigs of parsley
550ml/1 pint water

1 beef stock cube
3 × 15ml spoons/3 tablespoons
  skimmed milk
salt, pepper
freshly ground black pepper

Put the courgettes, onion, garlic and parsley into a saucepan,
add the water and crumble in the stock cube. Heat to boiling
point, reduce the heat, cover and simmer for 15 minutes.
Sieve, or process in a blender. Return to the pan and add the
milk, then simmer for a further 10 minutes. Season to taste,
and serve hot with a garnish of black pepper.

Serves 4

Total CHO   *20g*
Total calories *100*

Vegetable Soup

4 stalks celery, trimmed and chopped
100g/4 oz white cabbage, finely
  chopped
225g/8 oz courgettes, sliced
1 medium red pepper, deseeded and
  chopped

275ml/½ pint tomato juice
550ml/1 pint cold water
fresh parsley, chopped
1 chicken stock cube
50g/2 oz button mushrooms, sliced
salt, pepper

Put the celery, cabbage, courgettes and pepper into a large saucepan, add the tomato juice, water and parsley, then crumble in the stock cube. Heat to boiling point, reduce the heat, cover and simmer for 45 minutes. Ten minutes before the end of the cooking time, add the mushrooms. Season to taste, and garnish with a little chopped parsley.

Serves 4

Total CHO   **20g**
Total calories   **140**

Cock-a-Leekie

225g/8 oz courgettes, sliced
450g/1lb leeks, trimmed and sliced
1 large carrot, sliced
1 large onion, chopped
2 bay leaves
4 whole cloves

salt, freshly ground black pepper
550ml/1 pint cold water
1 chicken stock cube

Garnish
fresh parsley, chopped

Put the vegetables, bay leaves, cloves and seasoning in a saucepan. Add the water and crumble in the stock cube. Heat to boiling point, reduce the heat, cover and simmer for 45 minutes. Remove the bay leaves and cloves. Season to taste, and garnish with chopped parsley.

Serves 4

Total CHO   **40g**
Total calories   **180**

Thick Onion Soup (1)

3 large onions, sliced
2 large carrots, sliced
2 stalks celery, trimmed and chopped
550ml/1 pint cold water
1 × 2.5ml spoon/½ teaspoon ground
  nutmeg
1 chicken stock cube

salt, pepper
1 × 5ml spoon/1 teaspoon cornflour
50g/2 oz Edam cheese, grated

Accompaniment
triangles of toast from 1 large thin slice
  of wholemeal bread

Put the onions, carrots, celery and water into a large
saucepan. Add the nutmeg, crumble in the stock cube and
season to taste. Heat to boiling point, reduce the heat, cover
and simmer for 30 minutes.

Mix the cornflour with a little cold water and add to the
soup, stirring all the time until the soup thickens.

Pour the soup into bowls and top with the grated cheese.
Place under a hot grill for a few minutes or until the cheese
melts. Serve immediately with the triangles of toast.

Serves 4

Total CHO   ***60g***
Total calories ***480***

Thick Onion Soup (2)

3 large onions, chopped
2 medium tomatoes, chopped
1 large carrot, sliced
2 bay leaves
nutmeg
550ml/1 pint cold water

4 × 15ml spoons/4 tablespoons dry
  white wine
1 beef stock cube
1 × 5ml spoon/1 teaspoon arrowroot
salt, pepper
25g/1 oz Parmesan cheese, grated

Put the onions, tomatoes, carrot, bay leaves and nutmeg into
a saucepan. Add the water and wine, and crumble in the
stock cube. Heat to boiling point, reduce the heat, cover and
simmer for 30 minutes. Remove the bay leaves.

Mix the arrowroot with a little cold water and stir into the
soup to thicken it slightly. Simmer for a further 10 minutes,
then season to taste. Serve with the Parmesan cheese
sprinkled on the top.

Serves 4

Total CHO   ***40g***
Total calories ***320***

Iced Watercress Soup

2 bunches watercress, chopped
1 × 5ml spoon/1 teaspoon tarragon
550ml/1 pint cold water
1 chicken stock cube

3 × 15ml spoons/3 tablespoons
 skimmed milk
salt, pepper

Garnish
watercress leaves

Put the watercress and tarragon in a saucepan, add the
water and crumble in the stock cube. Heat to boiling point,
reduce the heat, cover and simmer for 20 minutes. Sieve, or
process in a blender. Return to the pan, add the milk and
simmer for a further 15 minutes. Season to taste and chill in a
refrigerator. Serve cold, and garnish with a few watercress
leaves.

Serves 4

Total CHO   *neg*
Total calories   *40*

Starters

Asparagus Snack

50g/2 oz button mushrooms, sliced
6 asparagus tips
3 × 15ml spoons/3 tablespoons
 skimmed milk
salt, pepper
2 large thin slices wholemeal bread

25g/1 oz Edam cheese, grated

Garnish
tomato slices
fresh parsley, chopped

Put the mushrooms, asparagus tips, skimmed milk and
seasoning in a saucepan and heat slowly for 10 minutes
stirring frequently.
   Toast the bread and top with the mushroom and asparagus
mixture. Sprinkle with the grated cheese, and grill for 2
minutes until melted. Garnish with the tomato slices and
chopped parsley. Serve immediately.

Serves 2

Total CHO   *30g*
Total calories *240*

Stuffed Red Peppers

2 large red peppers
25g/1 oz fresh wholemeal breadcrumbs
50g/2 oz Edam cheese, grated
1 medium onion, finely chopped
4 × 15ml spoons/4 tablespoons tomato
 juice

1 × 2.5ml spoon/½ teaspoon garlic salt
1 × 2.5ml spoon/½ teaspoon oregano
salt, pepper

Garnish
fresh parsley, chopped

Cut the peppers in half crossways and scoop out the seeds.
Cook in boiling salted water for 5 minutes, then drain well.
   Mix together the breadcrumbs, cheese, onion, tomato juice,
garlic salt and oregano. Season to taste, then divide the
stuffing into four and use to fill the peppers. Cover with foil
and cook at 190°C/375°F/Gas 5 for 25 minutes. Garnish
with the chopped parsley and serve hot or cold.

Serves 2

Total CHO   30g
Total calories 300

Cocktail Crevette

100g/4 oz curd cheese
150g/5.3 oz natural yoghurt (1 small
 carton)
100g/4 oz peeled shrimps
25g/1 oz chives, chopped
1 × 5ml spoon/1 teaspoon curry powder

lettuce, shredded

Garnish
cucumber slices
paprika

Mix together the curd cheese, yoghurt, shrimps, chives and
curry powder. Serve on a bed of shredded lettuce and garnish
with the cucumber slices and a sprinkling of paprika.

Serves 2
Total CHO   10g
Total calories 340

Melon Cheese

450g/1 lb cantaloupe melon, skinned,
 deseeded and cubed
100g/4 oz cottage cheese

juice of 1 lemon
½ medium apple, cored and chopped
ground cinnamon

Mix together all the ingredients except the cinnamon. Chill in
a refrigerator and sprinkle with cinnamon before serving.

Serves 2
Total CHO   20g
Total calories 200

Salmon Stuffed Eggs

2 size 3 eggs, hard-boiled
3 × 15ml spoons / 3 tablespoons natural
 yoghurt
1 × 75g/3 oz can salmon, drained
fresh parsley, chopped

salt, pepper

Garnish
sprigs of parsley

Cut the eggs in half crossways and carefully remove the
yolks. Mix with the yoghurt, salmon and parsley, then season
to taste. Use to fill the egg whites. Garnish with the sprigs of
parsley.

Serves 2

Total CHO   ***neg***
Total calories   ***240***

Pecan Melon Starter

$\frac{1}{2}$ small honeydew melon, skinned,
 deseeded and cubed
150g/5.3 oz natural yoghurt (1 small
 carton)

50g/2 oz pecan nuts, chopped
1 × 5ml spoon/1 teaspoon curry powder
lettuce, shredded
Cayenne pepper

Mix together the melon, yoghurt, nuts and curry powder. Pile
on to a bed of shredded lettuce and sprinkle with Cayenne
pepper. Chill well before serving.

Serves 2
Total CHO   ***30g***
Total calories   ***460***

Egg Pâté

2 size 3 eggs, hard-boiled
1 × 15ml spoon/1 tablespoon
 skimmed milk
paprika

salt, freshly ground black pepper
$\frac{1}{2}$ quantity of Slim Salad Sauce (page
 104)

Mash the eggs with a fork and add the remaining ingredients.
Process in a blender until smooth. Garnish with freshly ground
black pepper.

Serves 2
Total CHO   ***10g***
Total calories   ***200***

Serving suggestion Any green salad

Chilli Bean

75g/3 oz red kidney beans, dried **or**
  1 × 225g/8 oz can kidney beans,
  drained
1 small green pepper, deseeded and
  chopped
1 small red pepper, deseeded and
  chopped
2 fresh chillies, deseeded and sliced
1 × 5ml spoon/1 teaspoon English
  mustard powder
1 × 15ml spoon/1 tablespoon wine
  vinegar

1 × 5ml spoon/1 teaspoon olive oil
1 × 5ml spoon/1 teaspoon yeast extract
a dash of Tabasco sauce
1 clove of garlic, crushed
3 × 15ml spoons/3 tablespoons water
salt, pepper

Garnish
watercress

Soak the dried kidney beans overnight in water. Put in a pan
with sufficient salted water, bring rapidly to the boil, and boil
for 10 minutes. Reduce the heat, cover and simmer for a
further 50 minutes. Alternatively, cook in a pressure cooker.
Leave to cool, drain, then mix together with all the other
ingredients. Serve in a large salad bowl and garnish with the
watercress.

Serves 4

Total CHO   40g
Total calories 360

Ratatouille

2 × 5ml spoons/2 teaspoons vegetable
  oil
1 large aubergine, skinned and sliced
450g/1 lb courgettes, sliced
2 medium onions, chopped
100g/4 oz mushrooms, sliced
225g/8 oz tomatoes, skinned and
  chopped

3 × 15ml spoons/3 tablespoons
  tomato juice
100g/4 oz cauliflower florets
1 × 2.5ml spoon/$\frac{1}{2}$ teaspoon rosemary
1 × 2.5ml spoon/$\frac{1}{2}$ teaspoon basil
1 × 2.5ml spoon/$\frac{1}{2}$ teaspoon oregano
1 × 2.5ml spoon/$\frac{1}{2}$ teaspoon garlic salt
1 × 2.5ml spoon/$\frac{1}{2}$ teaspoon black
  pepper

Heat the oil in a non-stick pan. Gently fry the aubergine,
courgettes, onions and mushrooms for 10 minutes. Add the
tomatoes, tomato juice, cauliflower, herbs, garlic salt and
pepper, and cook for a further 15 minutes, stirring from time
to time.

Serves 4

Total CHO   40g
Total calories 240

Chinese Mushrooms

450g/1 lb button mushrooms
225g/8 oz bamboo shoots
225g/8 oz beansprouts
2 medium onions, finely chopped
1 medium leek, trimmed and finely sliced
1 × 5ml spoon/1 teaspoon ground
  ginger

2 × 15ml spoons/2 tablespoons soy
  sauce
275ml/½ pint cold water
1 chicken stock cube

Garnish
fresh chives, chopped
fresh parsley, chopped

Put the vegetables, ginger and soy sauce in a casserole. Add the water and crumble in the stock cube. Cook at 180°C/350°F/Gas 4 for 25 minutes. Garnish with the chives and parsley, and serve hot.

Serves 4

Total CHO   **20g**
Total calories   **140**

Mushrooms à la Grecque

450g/1lb button mushrooms, sliced

Marinade
juice of 1 lemon
150ml/¼ pint tomato juice
1 medium onion, chopped
1 × 15ml spoon/1 tablespoon fresh
  parsley, chopped
1 × 2.5ml spoon/½ teaspoon celery salt

1 × 2.5ml spoon/½ teaspoon thyme
1 × 2.5ml spoon/½ teaspoon coriander
  seeds
freshly ground black pepper

Garnish
fresh parsley, chopped

Make the marinade first. Mix all the ingredients together well, then leave to stand for 20 minutes.

   Add the mushrooms and pour into a casserole . Cook at 190°C/375°F/Gas 5 for 25 minutes. Garnish with the parsley, and serve hot or cold.

Serves 4

Total CHO   **10g**
Total calories   **60**

Mushrooms and Courgettes

450g/1 lb courgettes, sliced
225g/8 oz button mushrooms, sliced
1 medium onion, finely chopped
1 × 5ml spoon/1 teaspoon oregano
150ml/¼ pint cold water

1 beef stock cube
salt, pepper

Garnish
fresh chives, chopped

Put the courgettes, mushrooms, onion and oregano in a large saucepan, add the water and crumble in the stock cube. Heat to boiling point, reduce the heat, cover and simmer for 10 minutes. Remove the lid and simmer for a further 10 minutes until all the liquid is reduced. Garnish with the chives.

Serves 4

Total CHO   **20g**
Total calories   **140**

Sauerkraut with Ham

350g/12 oz sauerkraut
175g/6 oz cooked lean ham, cubed
100g/4 oz green peas, cooked
1 × 200g/7 oz can sweetcorn, drained

1 medium red pepper, deseeded and
  chopped
1 × 15ml spoon/1 tablespoon wine
  vinegar
salt, pepper

Mix all the ingredients together well and chill in a refrigerator before serving.

Serves 4
Total CHO   **40g**
Total calories   **460**

Chicken Liver Pâté

175g/6 oz chicken livers
1 large onion, finely chopped
1 × 5ml spoon/1 teaspoon curry powder
150ml/$\frac{1}{4}$ pint cold water
1 chicken stock cube
25g/1 oz fresh wholemeal breadcrumbs

juice of $\frac{1}{2}$ lemon
salt, pepper

Garnish
lemon slices

Put the liver, onion, curry powder and water in a saucepan, and crumble in the stock cube. Heat to boiling point, reduce the heat, cover and simmer for 15 minutes. Leave to cool slightly. Mix in the breadcrumbs, lemon juice, salt and pepper, then process in a blender until smooth. Pour into small pots and leave to chill in a refrigerator. Garnish with slices of lemon.

Serves 4

Total CHO   20g
Total calories 340

Calf's Liver Pâté

225g/8 oz calf's liver, sliced
1 small onion, finely chopped
2 cloves garlic, crushed
2 bay leaves
150ml/$\frac{1}{4}$ pint cold water
1 chicken stock cube
salt, pepper

juice of $\frac{1}{2}$ lemon
50g/2 oz curd cheese
50g/2 oz fresh wholemeal breadcrumbs

Garnish
fresh parsley, chopped

Put the liver, onion, garlic and bay leaves in a saucepan, add the water, crumble in the stock cube, and season to taste. Heat to boiling point, reduce the heat, cover and simmer for 20 minutes. Strain off the juice and stir in the lemon juice, curd cheese and breadcrumbs. Pour into small pots and chill in a refrigerator until set. Garnish with chopped parsley.

Serving suggestion Fingers of wholemeal toast

Serves 4

Total CHO   20g
Total calories 580

Mackerel Pâté

200g/7 oz smoked mackerel fillets, flaked
150g/5.3 oz natural yoghurt (1 small carton)

75g/3 oz fresh wholemeal breadcrumbs
2 cloves garlic, crushed
juice of 1 lemon
freshly ground black pepper

Mix all the ingredients together to form a paste, or process in a blender until smooth. Serve in individual ramekin dishes.

Serving suggestion Any side salad

Serves 4
Total CHO **40g**
Total calories **800**

Fish Salad

50g/2 oz crabmeat, flaked
50g/2 oz tuna fish, flaked
50g/2 oz salmon, flaked
50g/2 oz peeled prawns
6 stalks celery, trimmed and chopped
½ cucumber, peeled and cubed
100g/4 oz button mushrooms, sliced

juice of 1 lemon
1 × 5ml spoon/1 teaspoon celery salt
freshly ground black pepper

Garnish
lemon twists
tomato wedges

Mix together all the ingredients, and chill in a refrigerator for at least 2 hours before serving. Garnish with lemon twists and tomato wedges.

Serves 4
Total CHO **neg**
Total calories **280**

Crab Starter

2 × 15ml spoons/2 tablespoons wine vinegar
1 × 225g/8 oz can crabmeat, drained
2 medium onions, finely chopped
½ small cucumber, peeled and cubed
2 medium tomatoes, skinned and chopped
4 stalks celery, trimmed and chopped

150g/5.3 oz natural yoghurt (1 small carton)
1 red chilli, deseeded and sliced
4 black olives, stoned
fresh spinach, cooked and chopped

Garnish
red pepper, chopped

Mix together all the ingredients apart from the spinach. Pile the mixture on to a bed of spinach, then chill in a refrigerator. Garnish with chopped red pepper.

Serves 4
Total CHO **20g**
Total calories **460**

Hot Shrimp Savoury

225g/8 oz peeled shrimps
juice of 1 lemon
150g/5.3 oz natural yoghurt (1 small
  carton)
4 large thin slices wholemeal bread
2 size 3 egg whites

50g/2 oz Edam cheese, grated
salt, pepper

Garnish
watercress
thin tomato slices

Mix together the shrimps, lemon juice and yoghurt. Divide into four and use to cover each slice of bread. Whisk the egg whites until stiff, then fold in the cheese, and season to taste. Top each slice of bread with the mixture and cook at 190°C/375°F/Gas 5 for 20 minutes until the topping is golden-brown. Garnish with the watercress and tomato slices. Serve immediately.

Serves 4

Total CHO   60g
Total calories 800

Seafood Cocktail

1 × 100g/4 oz can crabmeat, drained
1 × 100g/4 oz can shrimps, drained
6 green peppercorns, crushed
½ quantity of Tomato Sauce (1)
  (page 105)

juice of 1 lemon

Garnish
shrimps
thin lemon slices

Mix together the crabmeat and shrimps. Add the crushed peppercorns to the tomato sauce and lemon juice, then mix with the seafood. Serve in glass dishes and garnish with a few shrimps and lemon slices.

Serves 4

Total CHO   10g
Total calories 200

Grapefruit and Prawns

350g/12 oz peeled prawns
2 large grapefruits, divided into
  segments
1 small onion, chopped
100g/4 oz cottage cheese

4 drops Tabasco sauce
25g/1 oz fresh parsley, chopped
salt, pepper
lettuce
paprika

Mix together the prawns, grapefruit, onion, cottage cheese, Tabasco sauce and parsley, and season to taste. Chill in a refrigerator. Serve on a bed of lettuce, and sprinkle with paprika.

Serves 4

Total CHO   20g
Total calories 580

Cottage-Celery Dip

225g/8 oz cottage cheese
150ml/¼ pint skimmed milk
1 medium onion, finely chopped
salt, pepper

Accompaniment
1 large head of celery, trimmed and
  separated

Pass the cheese and milk through a sieve, or process in a
blender until smooth. Add the onion, and season to taste.
Serve with the sticks of celery.

Serves 4
Total CHO   20g
Total calories 300

Orange Avocado

1 medium avocado pear, sliced
1 large orange, divided into segments
½ quantity of Yoghurt Dressing (2)
  (page 100)

1 Cos lettuce, chopped
Cayenne pepper

Mix together the avocado and orange segments, and gently
fold in the yoghurt dressing. Leave in a refrigerator to chill,
and serve on a bed of chopped lettuce. Sprinkle with
Cayenne pepper.

Serves 4

Total CHO   20g
Total calories 320

Grapefruit and Orange Cocktail

1 very large grapefruit, divided into
  segments
1 large orange, divided into segments
75ml/⅛ pint dry white wine

Garnish
sprigs of fresh mint

Marinate the fruit in the wine for at least 2 hours. Serve in
glass dishes garnished with sprigs of fresh mint.

Serves 4
Total CHO   20g
Total calories 120

31

Meat, Poultry and Game

It would be hard for most of us to imagine a diet which did not include meat and poultry. But, as they are concentrated sources of calories, the slimmer must get used to eating smaller quantities. You can, however, compensate for this by adding more vegetables, thereby satisfying both your diet sheet and your appetite.

The recipes in this chapter use chicken, rabbit or liver – all of which are relatively low in fat – as well as lean cuts of beef, pork and lamb.

To keep the calories down, fat is hardly ever added in the cooking and you should be sure always to trim the meat and skim the stock as thoroughly as possible.

Meat

Beef with Gherkin Sauce

225g/8 oz lean stewing beef, trimmed
  and cubed
1 medium onion, finely chopped
1 medium carrot, sliced
1 celery stalk, trimmed and chopped
150ml/¼ pint water
salt, pepper
1 × 5ml spoon/1 teaspoon mixed herbs

8 small gherkins
1 beef stock cube
150g/5.3 oz natural yoghurt (1 small
  carton)
25g/1 oz curd cheese

Garnish
chopped gherkins

Put the beef, onion, carrot, celery, water, seasoning, mixed herbs and gherkins in a large saucepan. Crumble in the stock cube. Heat slowly to boiling point, reduce the heat, cover and simmer for 1 hour. Cool slightly, season to taste and stir in the yoghurt and curd cheese. Serve immediately, garnished with chopped gherkins.

Serves 2

Total CHO   20g
Total calories 500

Serving suggestion Brown rice and green beans

Country Soup (page 18)

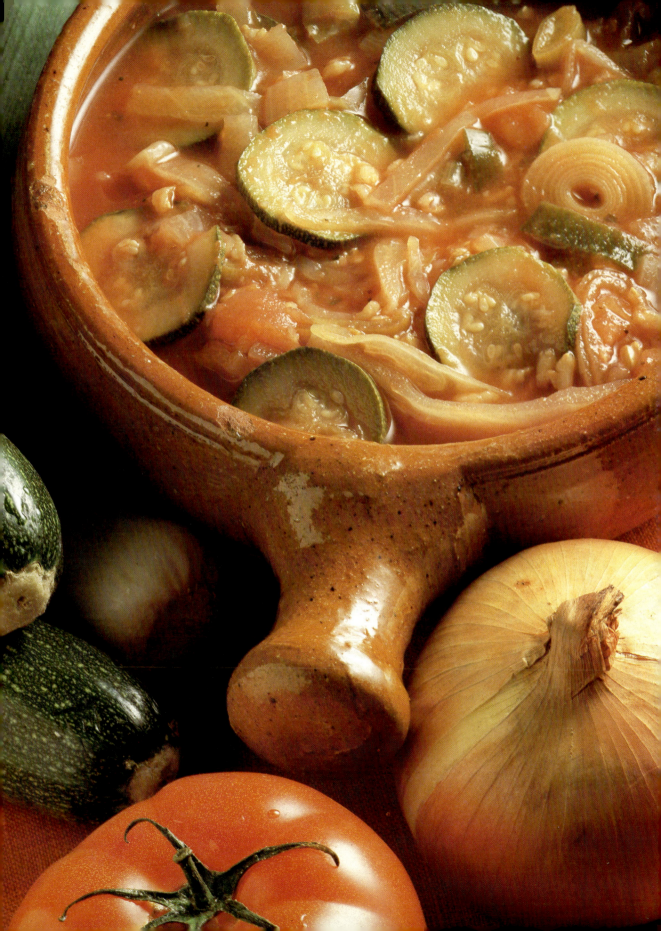

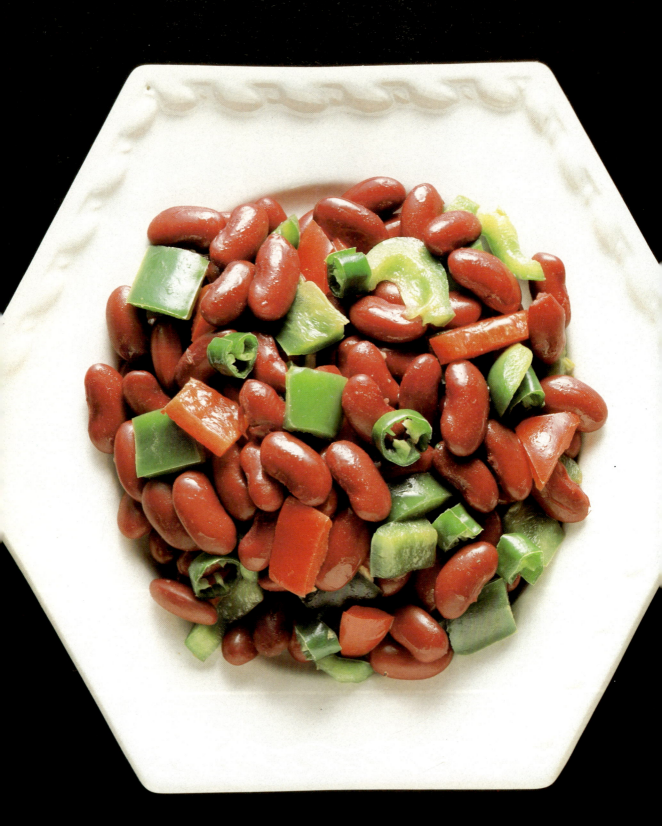

Bolognaise

225g/8 oz lean minced beef
1 medium onion, finely chopped
3 × 15ml spoons/3 tablespoons
  concentrated tomato purée
150ml/¼ pint water

1 × 2.5ml spoon/½ teaspoon parsley
1 × 2.5ml spoon/½ teaspoon thyme
1 × 2.5ml spoon/½ teaspoon oregano
salt, pepper

Heat a non-stick frying pan and add the beef, turning it
carefully to seal all sides. Transfer to a casserole with all the
other ingredients. Cook at 190°C/375°F/Gas 5 for 1 hour,
drain, then season to taste.

Serves 2

Total CHO   **10g**
Total calories   **480**

Serving suggestion Wholewheat pasta and green peas

Jarret of Veal

225g/8 oz fillet of veal
275ml/½ pint water
1 clove of garlic, crushed
2 × 15ml spoons/2 tablespoons
  concentrated tomato purée
parsley

1 chicken stock cube
salt, pepper
paprika
1 medium carrot, thinly sliced
2 stalks celery, trimmed and chopped
1 large tomato, skinned and sliced

Divide the meat into two portions, and cook under a hot grill
for 3 minutes on each side. Put in a casserole, add the water,
garlic, tomato purée and parsley, then crumble in the stock
cube, and season to taste. Leave to stand for 1 hour and then
add the vegetables. Cook at 220°C/425°F/Gas 7 for 20
minutes. Serve immediately.

Serves 2

Total CHO   **neg**
Total calories   **320**

Serving suggestion Wholewheat pasta and mixed vegetables

Chilli Bean (page 25)

Gouda Escalopes

2 small escalopes of veal (100g/4 oz each)
2 cloves garlic, crushed
1 × 2.5ml spoon/½ teaspoon celery salt
freshly ground black pepper

1 × 5ml spoon/1 teaspoon capers, chopped
2 × 15ml spoons/2 tablespoons tomato juice
50g/2 oz Gouda cheese, thinly sliced

Put the escalopes in a casserole. Rub over with the crushed garlic and then sprinkle with the celery salt, pepper, capers and tomato juice. Cover and leave to stand for 2 hours. Place the cheese over the meat, and cook at 220°C/425°F/Gas 7 for 25 minutes.

Serves 2

Total CHO   **neg**
Total calories   **420**

Serving suggestion Jacket potatoes and butter beans

Navarin of Veal

225g/8 oz fillet of veal, cubed
275ml/½ pint water
½ chicken stock cube
1 medium onion, finely chopped
2 stalks celery, trimmed and chopped
2 medium carrots, chopped
150ml/¼ pint tomato juice

1 × 15ml spoon/1 tablespoon Worcestershire sauce
salt, pepper

Garnish
100g/4 oz whole French beans

Mix together all the ingredients except for the green beans. Put in a casserole, and cook at 220°C/425°F/Gas 7 for 25 minutes.
    Cook the green beans in boiling salted water and use to garnish the veal when serving.

Serves 2

Total CHO   **10g**
Total calories   **320**

Serving suggestion Creamed potatoes and sweetcorn

Veal Casserole

225g/8 oz lean stewing veal, cubed
2 medium onions, finely chopped
2 medium green peppers, deseeded and
  chopped
225g/8 oz mushrooms, sliced
275ml/½ pint tomato juice

1 clove of garlic, crushed
1 × 15ml spoon/1 tablespoon soy sauce
1 × 5ml spoon/1 teaspoon oregano
salt, pepper
225g/8 oz whole green beans

Put all the ingredients except for the green beans in a
casserole. Cook at 190°C/375°F/Gas 5 for 1 hour. Add the
green beans and cook for a further 15 minutes. Serve hot.

Serves 2
Total CHO   30g
Total calories 400

Veal Cutlets with Mushroom Sauce

100g/4 oz button mushrooms
12 button onions
1 × 5ml spoon/1 teaspoon basil
1 × 5ml spoon/1 teaspoon celery salt
1 × 5ml spoon/1 teaspoon black pepper
275ml/½ pint water
1 chicken stock cube
2 veal cutlets (175g/6 oz each approx)

150g/5.3 oz natural yoghurt (1 small
  carton)
1 × 15ml spoon/1 tablespoon
  Worcestershire sauce

Garnish
fresh parsley, chopped

Put the mushrooms, onions, basil, celery salt and pepper in a
saucepan, add the water and crumble in the stock cube. Heat
to boiling point, reduce the heat, cover and simmer for 10
minutes. Put the veal cutlets into the stock and simmer for a
further 15 minutes, turning from time to time. When cooked,
stir in the yoghurt and Worcestershire sauce. Serve
immediately with a garnish of chopped parsley.

Serves 2

Total CHO   10g
Total calories 500

Serving suggestion Whole new potatoes and spinach

Stuffed Cutlets of Pork

2 medium pork cutlets, trimmed
1 clove of garlic, crushed
salt, pepper
1 large cooking apple, peeled, cored and
  sliced
1 small onion, finely chopped

150ml/¼ pint water
1 chicken stock cube
50g/2 oz brown rice, cooked

Garnish
chopped tomato

Rub the pork cutlets with the garlic. Sprinkle with salt and
pepper and grill gently for about 15 minutes on either side.
    Meanwhile, put the apple and onion in a saucepan, add the
water and crumble in the stock cube. Cook for 10 minutes.
Drain off any excess liquid, stir in the cooked rice, and season
to taste. Use this mixture to top each pork cutlet. Place on a
baking tray, cover with foil, and cook at 160°C/325°F/Gas 3
for 25 minutes. Garnish with chopped tomato.

Serving suggestion Cabbage and sweetcorn

Serves 2

Total CHO   **60g**
Total calories **700**

Pork Rissoles

175g/6 oz lean pork, minced
25g/1 oz fresh wholemeal breadcrumbs
1 × 5ml spoon/1 teaspoon made
  French mustard
1 × 5ml spoon/1 teaspoon
  concentrated tomato purée

1 clove of garlic, crushed
salt, pepper

Garnish
fresh parsley, chopped
tomato slices

Mix all the ingredients together well, and form into two
rissoles. Grill under a medium heat for ten minutes on each
side. Garnish with chopped parsley and tomato slices.

Serving suggestion Green salad and wholemeal rolls

Serves 2
Total CHO   **10g**
Total calories **320**

Calf's Liver With Fennel

1 bulb of fennel, trimmed and sliced
1 medium green pepper, deseeded and
  chopped
100g/4 oz mushrooms, sliced
150ml/¼ pint water
salt, pepper

2 × 5ml spoons/2 teaspoons mixed
  herbs
1 clove of garlic, crushed
1 chicken stock cube
225g/8 oz calf's liver, sliced
juice of ½ lemon

Put the vegetables in a large saucepan. Add the water,
seasoning, herbs and garlic, and crumble in the stock cube.
Heat to boiling point, reduce the heat, cover and simmer for
20 minutes. Dip the liver in the lemon juice and grill for 8
minutes on each side. Transfer to a serving dish and cover
with the vegetables. Serve immediately.

Serves 2

Total CHO   10g
Total calories 440

Spiced Liver

225g/8 oz lamb's liver, thinly sliced
2 medium tomatoes, chopped
1 medium onion, finely chopped
1 medium green pepper, deseeded and
  chopped
1 medium courgette, sliced
150ml/¼ pint water

1 × 2.5ml spoon/½ teaspoon paprika
salt, pepper
1 clove of garlic, crushed
1 beef stock cube

Garnish
fresh parsley, chopped

Put the liver and vegetables in a large saucepan. Add the
water, paprika, salt, pepper and garlic, and crumble in the
stock cube. Heat to boiling point, reduce the heat, cover and
simmer for 30 minutes. Garnish with chopped parsley.

Serves 2

Total CHO   10g
Total calories 480

Rich Beef Casserole

1 × 5ml spoon/1 teaspoon vegetable oil
275g/10 oz stewing beef, trimmed and
  cubed
1 × 15ml spoon/1 tablespoon
  concentrated tomato purée
2 medium carrots, sliced
2 medium onions, sliced

2 medium tomatoes, chopped
275ml/½ pint water
2 cloves garlic, crushed
fresh parsley, chopped
1 beef stock cube
salt, pepper

Serves 4

Heat the oil in a non-stick frying pan and add the beef, turning
it carefully to seal all sides. Stir in the tomato purée, and add
the vegetables. Heat to boiling point, and then transfer to a
casserole. Add the water, garlic and parsley, crumble in the
stock cube, and season to taste. Cook at 190°C/375°F/Gas
5 for 1 hour.

Total CHO   20g
Total calories   560

Serving suggestion Jacket potatoes and spring greens

Sweet and Sour Meatballs

350g/12 oz lean minced beef
1 small onion
75g/3 oz fresh wholemeal breadcrumbs
salt, pepper
1 size 3 egg, well beaten
150ml/¼ pint water
1 beef stock cube
2 stalks celery, trimmed and chopped
1 medium carrot, finely sliced

1 small leek, finely sliced
1 medium onion, trimmed and finely
  chopped
4 × 15ml spoons/4 tablespoons vinegar
2 × 15ml spoons/2 tablespoons
  concentrated tomato purée
2 × 15ml spoons/2 tablespoons soy
  sauce
liquid sweetener

Serves 4

Mix together the minced beef, onion, breadcrumbs, salt and
pepper, and bind together with the beaten egg. Form the
mixture into small balls. Put the remaining ingredients, except
the liquid sweetener, in a saucepan, heat to boiling point,
reduce the heat, cover and simmer for 10 minutes. Add the
meatballs and simmer for a further 15 minutes. Season to
taste, add the sweetener, and serve immediately.

Total CHO   40g
Total calories   960

Serving suggestion Wholewheat ribbon noodles and
broccoli

Meatballs with Green Pepper Sauce

450g/1 lb lean minced beef
1 size 3 egg, well beaten
100g/4 oz fresh wholemeal
  breadcrumbs
1 × 5ml spoon/1 teaspoon mixed dried
  herbs
425ml/¾ pint boiling water
1 beef stock cube
salt, pepper

Green Pepper Sauce
275ml/½ pint skimmed milk
1 × 15ml spoon/1 tablespoon arrowroot
1 × 15ml spoon/1 tablespoon low fat
  margarine
½ small green pepper, deseeded and
  chopped
1 × 5ml spoon/1 teaspoon soy sauce
salt, pepper

Mix together the minced beef, egg, breadcrumbs and herbs. Leave to stand for 1 hour and then form the mixture into small balls. Put the water into a saucepan, crumble in the stock cube, add the meatballs, and season to taste. Heat to boiling point, reduce the heat, cover and simmer for 30 minutes.

Meanwhile, make the sauce. Put the milk, arrowroot and margarine into a saucepan. Heat slowly to boiling point, stirring all the time. Reduce the heat, add the green pepper and soy sauce, and season to taste. Simmer for a further 5 minutes, stirring from time to time.

Remove the meatballs from the stock, pour the sauce over them, and serve immediately.

Serving suggestion Wholewheat ribbon noodles and green beans

Serves 4

Total CHO   80g
Total calories 1260

Hot Lamb Curry

2 × 5ml spoons/2 teaspoons vegetable
  oil
450g/1 lb lean lamb, cut into small
  cubes
3 medium onions, chopped
2 cloves garlic, crushed
25g/1 oz lentils
1 × 5ml spoon/1 teaspoon curry paste
1 × 5ml spoon/1 teaspoon Cayenne
  pepper
1 × 2.5ml spoon/½ teaspoon cardamon
1 × 2.5ml spoon/½ teaspoon coriander
  seeds

1 × 2.5ml spoon/½ teaspoon cinnamon
25g/1 oz fresh root ginger
150ml/¼ pint water
juice of 1 lemon
1 chicken stock cube
100g/4 oz frozen peas
salt, pepper
150g/5.3 oz natural yoghurt (1 small
  carton)

Garnish
lemon slices

Heat the oil in a non-stick saucepan and add the lamb, turning it carefully to seal all sides. Add the onions and garlic and cook until the onion is soft. Stir in the lentils and spices, then add the water and lemon juice, and crumble in the stock cube. Heat to boiling point, reduce the heat, cover and simmer for 1 hour. Add the peas and remove the piece of ginger 5 minutes before serving. Season to taste, and stir in the yoghurt. Serve garnished with lemon slices.

Serves 4

Total CHO   40g
Total calories 1100

Serving suggestion Brown rice and any side salad

Ragoût of Lamb

1 clove of garlic
450g/1 lb lean stewing lamb, cubed
2 medium onions, finely chopped
1 × 2.5ml spoon/½ teaspoon rosemary
1 × 2.5ml spoon/½ teaspoon basil

salt, pepper
275ml/½ pint water
1 chicken stock cube
175g/6 oz broad beans, lightly cooked

Rub the garlic over the lamb. Mix together the lamb, onions and herbs, season to taste, and leave to stand for 30 minutes in a casserole. Add the water, crumble in the stock cube, and cook at 200°C/400°F/Gas 6 for 1 hour. Five minutes before serving, stir in the broad beans.

Serves 4

Total CHO   20g
Total calories 860

Serving suggestion Jacket potatoes and mixed vegetables

Indian Lamb Kebabs

1 × 5ml spoon/1 teaspoon turmeric
1 × 5ml spoon/1 teaspoon paprika
1 × 5ml spoon/1 teaspoon celery salt
2 × 5ml spoons/2 teaspoons vegetable
  oil
4 × 15ml spoons/4 tablespoons wine
  vinegar
juice of 1 lemon
2 bay leaves

liquid sweetener
450g/1 lb fillet of lamb, cut into
  2.5cm/1 inch cubes
100g/4 oz button mushrooms

Garnish
tomato slices
watercress

Put the turmeric, paprika, celery salt, oil, vinegar, lemon juice, bay leaves and the liquid sweetener in a bowl and mix well. Add the lamb, and marinate for 4 hours, turning from time to time.

Thread the meat on to long skewers, alternating with the mushrooms, Grill for about 10 minutes on each side, until well browned and cooked through, brushing several times with the marinade. Garnish with tomato slices and watercress.

Serving suggestion Brown rice and any mixed salad

Serves 4

Total CHO   neg
Total calories 860

Mustard Pork and Mushrooms

1 × 15ml spoon/1 tablespoon made
  English mustard
2 × 15ml spoons/2 tablespoons
  concentrated tomato purée
350g/12 oz lean pork fillet, cubed
1 × 425g/15 oz can butter beans,
  drained

150ml/$\frac{1}{4}$ pint tomato juice
100g/4 oz button mushrooms, sliced
1 × 2.5ml spoon/$\frac{1}{2}$ teaspoon rosemary
1 × 2.5ml spoon/$\frac{1}{2}$ teaspoon thyme
1 × 2.5ml spoon/$\frac{1}{2}$ teaspoon garlic salt
1 × 2.5ml spoon/$\frac{1}{2}$ teaspoon black
  pepper

Mix together the mustard and tomato purée, and use to coat the pork. Place in an ovenproof dish. Add the remaining ingredients, cover with foil, seal well and cook at 190°C/375°F/Gas 5 for 40 minutes.

Serving suggestion Jacket potatoes and green peas

Serves 4

Total CHO   60g
Total calories 860

Liver Kebabs

150ml/¼ pint water
1 beef stock cube
225g/8 oz lamb's liver, cubed
8 small gherkins

50g/2 oz Edam cheese, cubed
4 slices pineapple, cubed
lettuce

Put the water in a saucepan, crumble in the stock cube and add the liver. Cook for about 15 minutes. Leave to cool completely and arrange on cocktail sticks with the other ingredients. Serve on a bed of lettuce.

Serves 4

Total CHO   **20g**
Total calories 640

Liver Casserole

450g/1 lb pig's liver
100g/4 oz mushrooms, sliced
4 stalks celery, trimmed and chopped
1 large onion, chopped
1 clove of garlic, crushed
1 bay leaf
1 × 5ml spoon/1 teaspoon basil

salt, pepper
275ml/½ pint water
1 beef stock cube

Garnish
fresh parsley, chopped

Put the liver in a large casserole with the vegetables, herbs and seasoning. Add the water and crumble in the stock cube, then cook at 180°C/350°F/Gas 4 for 1¼ hours. Remove the bay leaf and serve with a garnish of chopped parsley.

Serves 4

Total CHO   **10g**
Total calories 780

Poultry and Game

Pineapple Chicken

2 chicken breasts, skinned and boned
150ml/¼ pint pineapple juice
2 slices canned pineapple in natural
  juice, chopped
2 × 15ml spoons/2 tablespoons dry
  white wine

1 × 2.5ml spoon/½ teaspoon garlic salt
freshly ground black pepper

Garnish
sprigs of watercress
tomato slices

Put all the ingredients in a casserole, cover and leave in a refrigerator to marinate overnight. Cook at 180°C/350°F/Gas 4 for 30 minutes. Garnish with watercress and tomato slices.

Serves 2
Total CHO   **30g**
Total calories 380

Sherry Chicken

2 chicken breasts, skinned and boned
juice of 2 lemons and grated rind of 1
  lemon
1 × 5ml spoon/1 teaspoon vegetable oil
1 medium carrot, sliced
3 medium onions, chopped
1 medium red pepper, deseeded and
  chopped
225g/8 oz white cabbage, shredded

2 × 15ml spoons/2 tablespoons dry
  sherry
2 × 15ml spoons/2 tablespoons wine
  vinegar
1 × 5ml spoon/1 teaspoon ground
  ginger
salt, pepper

Garnish
fresh chives, chopped

Flatten out the chicken breasts with a rolling-pin. Sprinkle with half the lemon juice and leave to stand for 1 hour. Heat the oil in a pan and gently cook the carrot, onions, pepper and cabbage until soft. Stir in the sherry, vinegar, remaining lemon juice, lemon rind, ginger, salt and pepper, and cook for a further 2 minutes. Place the chicken in an ovenproof dish and spread the cooked vegetables on top. Cover with foil and cook at 190°C/375°F/Gas 5 for 30 minutes. Garnish with chopped chives.

Serving suggestion Whole new potatoes and whole green beans

Serves 2

Total CHO   ***30g***
Total calories ***460***

Citrus Chicken

225g/8 oz cooked chicken, diced
75ml/$\frac{1}{8}$ pint unsweetened orange juice
juice and grated rind of 1 lemon
1 medium onion, chopped
1 medium red pepper, deseeded and
  chopped

thyme
salt, pepper
225g/8 oz white cabbage, shredded

Put the chicken in a saucepan with the orange juice, lemon juice, lemon rind, onion, red pepper and thyme. Season to taste, and simmer for 15 minutes. Fold the cabbage into the chicken mixture, cover and cook for a further 2 minutes. Serve immediately with soy sauce.

Serving suggestion Brown rice and mixed vegetables

Serves 2

Total CHO   ***20g***
Total calories ***440***

Turkey Courgettes

225g/8 oz turkey, cubed
450g/1 lb courgettes, sliced
1 × 15ml spoon/1 tablespoon tomato
 juice
2 × 15ml spoons/2 tablespoons
 Worcestershire sauce
150ml/¼ pint water

1 chicken stock cube
1 medium onion, finely chopped
2 × 5ml spoons/2 teaspoons mixed
 herbs

Garnish
fresh parsley, chopped

Put all the ingredients in a casserole and cook at
190°C/375°F/Gas 5 for 30 minutes. Garnish with chopped
parsley and serve immediately.

Serves 2
Total CHO   ***20g***
Total calories   ***420***

Serving suggestion Whole new potatoes and spinach

Turkey Seconds

2 medium onions, chopped
100g/4 oz button mushrooms
25g/1 oz fresh parsley, chopped
½ small cucumber, peeled and cubed
juice of 1 lemon
150ml/¼ pint water
1 chicken stock cube
225g/8 oz cooked turkey, finely chopped

1 × 15ml spoon/1 tablespoon skimmed
 milk
1 × 5ml spoon/1 teaspoon celery salt
pepper

Garnish
fresh mushrooms, chopped

Put the onions, mushrooms, parsley, cucumber and lemon
juice in a saucepan. Add the water and crumble in the stock
cube. Heat to boiling point, reduce the heat, cover and
simmer for 10 minutes. Add the turkey and simmer for a
further 20 minutes. Remove from the heat, then add the milk
and salt and pepper to taste. Serve with a garnish of chopped
mushrooms.

Serves 2

Total CHO   ***10g***
Total calories   ***400***

Serving suggestion Brown rice and green peas

Spicy Rabbit

225g/8 oz rabbit meat, minced
1 large onion, finely chopped
2 medium tomatoes, skinned and
  chopped
1 medium green pepper, deseeded and
  chopped
1 medium red pepper, deseeded and
  chopped
150ml/$\frac{1}{4}$ pint water
1 chicken stock cube

1 clove of garlic, crushed
1 × 2.5ml spoon/$\frac{1}{2}$ teaspoon rosemary
1 × 2.5ml spoon/$\frac{1}{2}$ teaspoon ground
  ginger
1 × 2.5ml spoon/$\frac{1}{2}$ teaspoon cinnamon
salt, pepper

Garnish
nutmeg

Mix all the ingredients together well and put in a casserole.
Cook at 190°C/375°F/Gas 5 for 25 minutes. Transfer to a
serving dish, sprinkle with nutmeg and serve immediately.

Serves 2
Total CHO   **20g**
Total calories 400

Serving suggestion Brown rice and carrots

Marinated Chicken Casserole

4 chicken breasts, skinned and boned
275ml/$\frac{1}{2}$ pint cold water
juice of 1 lemon
1 chicken stock cube
1 × 15ml spoon/1 tablespoon sunflower
  oil
2 medium onions, sliced
1 medium green pepper, deseeded and
  sliced

100g/4 oz button mushrooms, sliced
1 × 5ml spoon/1 teaspoon celery salt
1 × 5ml spoon/1 teaspoon paprika
1 × 5ml spoon/1 teaspoon coriander
  seeds
freshly ground black pepper

Put the chicken breasts, water and lemon juice in a casserole,
crumble in the stock cube, and marinate for 2 hours. Heat the
oil in a frying pan and gently cook the onions, pepper and
mushrooms until tender. Add the celery salt, paprika,
coriander seeds and pepper to taste, and cook for a further 2
minutes. Put the vegetable mixture into the casserole and
cook at 190°C/375°F/Gas 5 for 30 minutes.

Serves 4

Total CHO   **neg**
Total calories 700

Serving suggestion Jacket potatoes and green peas

Chicken Chasseur

4 medium carrots, sliced
2 medium onions, sliced
225g/8 oz button mushrooms, sliced
275ml/½ pint tomato juice
2 cloves garlic, crushed
150ml/¼ pint water
1 × 5ml spoon/1 teaspoon basil

salt, pepper
1 chicken stock cube
4 chicken breasts, skinned and boned
75g/3 oz sweetcorn
150g/5.3 oz natural yoghurt (1 small carton)

Put the carrots, onions, mushrooms, tomato juice and garlic in a large casserole. Add the water, basil and seasoning, and crumble in the stock cube. Cook at 180°C/350°F/Gas 4 for 45 minutes. Add the chicken pieces and sweetcorn, and cook for a further 30 minutes. Place the chicken on a hot serving dish. Stir the yoghurt into the sauce in the casserole, then pour it over the chicken and serve immediately.

Serves 4

Total CHO   60g
Total calories 880

Serving suggestion Jacket potatoes and green peas

Chicken Paprika

4 small chicken legs, skinned
2 × 5ml spoons/2 teaspoons paprika
150ml/¼ pint water
1 chicken stock cube
1 small onion, finely chopped
1 medium red pepper, deseeded and chopped

1 medium green pepper, deseeded and chopped
1 clove of garlic, crushed
salt, pepper

Garnish
paprika

Put all the ingredients in a casserole and cook at 200°C/400°F/Gas 6 for 40 minutes. Place the chicken in a serving dish and pour over the liquid. Garnish with a sprinkling of paprika.

Serves 4

Total CHO   neg
Total calories 480

Serving suggestion Jacket potatoes and sweetcorn

Coq au Vin

4 chicken breasts, skinned and boned
150ml/¼ pint dry white wine
100g/4 oz button mushrooms, sliced
1 medium carrot, sliced
1 medium onion, chopped
1 × 5ml spoon/1 teaspoon oregano

salt, pepper
150ml/¼ pint water
1 chicken stock cube

Garnish
fresh parsley, chopped

Put the chicken, wine, vegetables, oregano, salt and pepper in a large casserole. Add the water and crumble in the stock cube. Cook at 180°C/350°F/Gas 4 for 40 minutes. Serve with a garnish of chopped parsley.

Serves 4

Total CHO **10g**
Total calories **680**

Chinatown Rabbit

450g/1 lb rabbit meat, cubed
450g/1 lb beansprouts
225g/8 oz bamboo shoots, chopped
3 medium onions, finely chopped
225g/8 oz whole French green beans
225g/8 oz white cabbage, finely
  shredded
275ml/½ pint water

2 × 15ml spoons/2 tablespoons
  Worcestershire sauce
1 × 15ml spoon/1 tablespoon
  concentrated tomato purée
2 cloves garlic, crushed
2 × 5ml spoons/2 teaspoons oregano
salt, pepper
1 chicken stock cube

Mix together the meat and vegetables. Add the water, Worcestershire sauce, tomato purée, garlic, oregano, salt and pepper, then crumble in the stock cube. Mix well and put in a casserole. Cook at 180°C/350°F/Gas 4 for 40 minutes. Serve with a dash of soy sauce.

Serves 4

Total CHO **40g**
Total calories **820**

Serving suggestion Brown rice and cauliflower

Fish and Shellfish

Fish and shellfish make an ideal main course. Every bit as delicious as meat, both contain less fat and therefore less calories. They are also excellent value for money as they shrink very little during cooking.

The recipes given here use just a few types of fish and shellfish, all of which are easily obtainable everywhere. But fishmongers offer an enormous variety of species from which to choose and you will have great fun selecting from amongst the broad range available.

Fish

Fish Curry

350g/12 oz cod steak
150ml/¼ pint fish stock (page 64)
2 medium onions, finely chopped
1 medium cooking apple, cored and
  chopped
juice of 1 lemon

1 × 5ml spoon/1 teaspoon curry powder
1 × 5ml spoon/1 teaspoon celery salt
freshly ground black pepper
100g/4 oz frozen peas
2 × 15ml spoons/2 tablespoons
  skimmed milk

Put the cod steak in a saucepan and add the stock, onions, apple, lemon juice, curry powder, celery salt and black pepper. Heat to boiling point, reduce the heat, cover and simmer for 30 minutes. Remove the lid, add the peas and cook for a further 10 minutes to reduce the liquid. Stir in the skimmed milk and serve immediately.

Serves 2

Total CHO   **30g**
Total calories **360**

Serving suggestion Brown rice and a selection of chutneys

*Indian Lamb Kebabs (page 43) with Brown rice and
Cucumber and Onion Raita (page 95)*

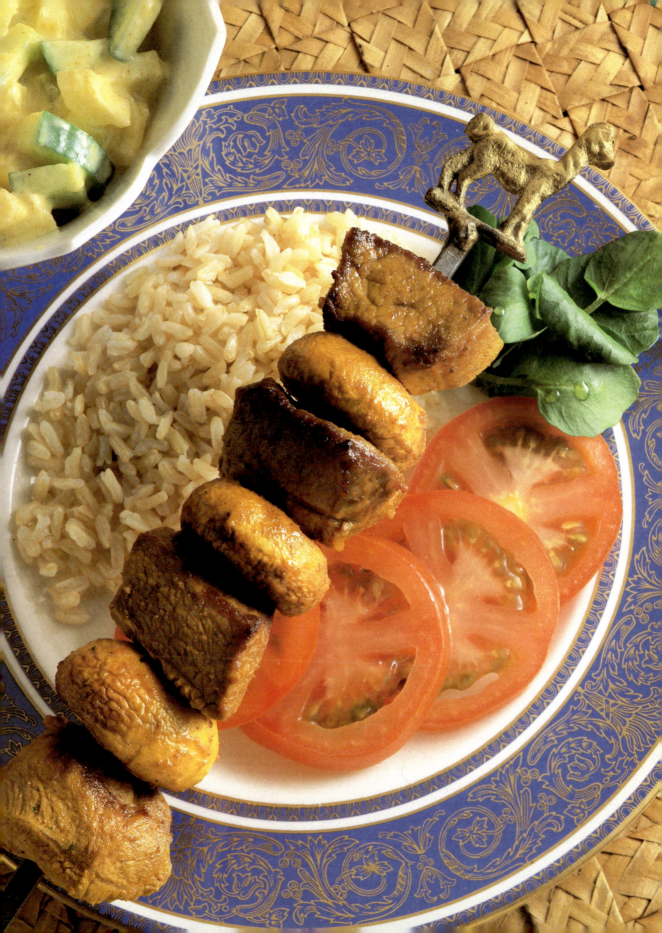

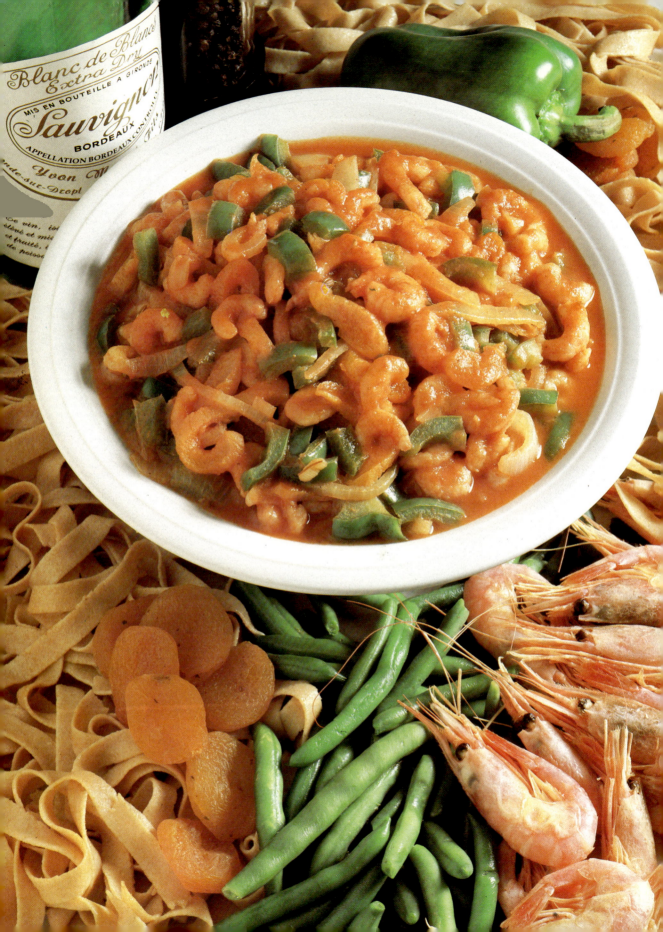

French Cod

2 medium onions, finely chopped
2 medium tomatoes, chopped
2 × 15ml spoons/2 tablespoons dry
  white wine
150ml/¼ pint water
1 bay leaf
1 clove of garlic, crushed
fresh parsley, chopped

1 × 5ml spoon/1 teaspoon celery salt
1 × 5ml spoon/1 teaspoon chopped
  chives
freshly ground black pepper
350g/12 oz cod fillet, cubed

Garnish
tomato slices

Put all the ingredients except the fish in a large saucepan.
Heat to boiling point, reduce the heat, cover and simmer for
10 minutes. Add the fish and simmer for a further 10 minutes.
Garnish with tomato slices.

Serves 2

Total CHO   *10g*
Total calories *320*

Serving suggestion Mashed potatoes and sweetcorn

Mariner's Cod

350g/12 oz cod steak
1 medium onion, finely chopped
1 clove of garlic, crushed
4 × 15ml spoons/4 tablespoons
  concentrated tomato purée
150ml/¼ pint water
100g/4 oz whole French green beans

1 × 2.5ml spoon/½ teaspoon celery salt
1 × 2.5ml spoon/½ teaspoon basil
freshly ground black pepper

Garnish
fresh parsley, chopped

Cut the fish into two pieces and put in a casserole with the
other ingredients. Cook at 220°C/425°F/Gas 7 for 20
minutes. Garnish with chopped parsley.

Serves 2
Total CHO   *10g*
Total calories *320*

Serving suggestion Wholewheat ribbon noodles and spinach

Pepper Prawns (page 62)

Cod-a-Leekie

225g/8 oz cod fillet
225g/8 oz leeks, trimmed and sliced
juice of 1 lemon

1 × 15ml spoon/1 tablespoon tomato
 juice
salt, pepper
150ml/¼ pint cold water

Put the fish in a casserole, and add the leeks, lemon juice, tomato juice, seasoning and water. Cover and cook at 190°C/375°F/Gas 5 for about 25 minutes.

Serves 2
Total CHO   neg
Total calories 200

Serving suggestion Jacket potatoes and carrots

Slimmer's Fish Cakes

350g/12 oz cod fillet, cooked and
 skinned
1 medium onion, finely chopped
1 × 15ml spoon/1 tablespoon
 Worcestershire sauce

1 × 5ml spoon/1 teaspoon made French
 mustard
fresh parsley, chopped
salt, pepper
1 size 3 egg, well beaten
1 × 5ml spoon/1 teaspoon vegetable oil

Mix together all the ingredients except the oil. Form into four round cakes and flatten. Heat the oil in a non-stick frying pan and cook the fish cakes slowly for 10 minutes on each side.

Serves 2
Total CHO   neg
Total calories 340

Serving suggestion Wholemeal baps and baked beans

Cidered Mackerel

2 small whole mackerel, ready gutted
juice of 1 lemon
1 large onion, finely chopped
1 bay leaf
salt, pepper
150ml/¼ pint dry cider

Garnish
fresh parsley, chopped

Accompaniment
stewed apple

Place the mackerel in a casserole with all the other ingredients and cook at 160°C/325°F/Gas 3 for 1 hour. Remove the bay leaf, garnish with chopped parsley and serve with a little stewed apple.

Serves 2

Total CHO   10g
Total calories 560

Serving suggestion Jacket potatoes and broccoli

Cold Fish Curls

225g/8 oz fillet of plaice
1 × 15ml spoon/1 tablespoon dry white
  wine
1 bay leaf
150ml/¼ pint fish stock (page 64)
½ medium red pepper, deseeded and
  chopped
½ medium green pepper, deseeded
  and chopped

1 small onion, finely chopped
parsley
salt, pepper
lettuce

Garnish
cucumber slices
lemon slices

Divide the fillet into two strips. Roll up each piece with the skin
on the inside and secure with cocktail sticks. Place in a
casserole with the remaining ingredients, except the lettuce.
Cover, and leave to stand for 2 hours. Cook at
190°C/375°F/Gas 5 for 20 minutes, then cool completely.
Serve on a bed of lettuce and garnish with slices of
cucumber and lemon.

Serving suggestion Cold wholewheat ribbon noodles and
any side salad

Serves 2

Total CHO   **neg**
Total calories   **240**

Party Fish Platter

350g/12 oz fillet of plaice
2 × 5ml spoons/2 teaspoons water
1 × 5ml spoon/1 teaspoon tarragon
salt, pepper
4 black olives

Garnish
thin lemon slices
fresh parsley, chopped

Divide the fillet into two strips. Roll up each piece with the skin
on the inside and secure with cocktail sticks. Put in an
ovenproof dish with the water, tarragon, salt and pepper.
Cover with foil and bake at 160°C/325°F/Gas 3 for about 20
minutes. Leave to cool completely. Place on a serving dish
with an olive at either end of each fillet. Garnish with lemon
slices and chopped parsley.

Serving suggestion Cold brown rice and bean salad

Serves 2

Total CHO   **neg**
Total calories   **320**

Curried Lemon Sole

2 fillets of lemon sole (175g/6 oz each)
2 × 15ml spoons/2 tablespoons dry
  white wine
juice of 1 lemon
5 × 15ml spoons/5 tablespoons water

1 × 5ml spoon/1 teaspoon curry powder
150g/5.3 oz natural yoghurt (1 small
  carton)
salt, pepper

Put the fish in a casserole. Mix together the wine, lemon juice, water, curry powder, yoghurt, salt and pepper. Pour the mixture over the fish, and cook at 190°C/375°F/Gas 5 for 25 minutes.

Serving suggestion Whole new potatoes and broccoli

Serves 2

Total CHO   10g
Total calories 380

Tarragon Sole

50g/2 oz button mushrooms
1 small onion, finely chopped
1 medium green pepper, deseeded
  and finely chopped
1 × 15ml spoon/1 tablespoon wine
  vinegar
150ml/¼ pint water
tarragon

parsley
salt, pepper
2 whole lemon sole, ready gutted (175-
  225g/6-8 oz each)

Garnish
lemon wedges
tomato wedges

Put the vegetables, vinegar, water, herbs, salt and pepper into an ovenproof dish. Place the fish, whole, on top and cover with foil. Cook at 180°C/350°F/Gas 4 for 25 minutes. Put the fish on a serving dish, drain the vegetables and arrange them around the fish. Garnish with lemon and tomato wedges.

Serving suggestion Jacket potatoes and sweetcorn

Serves 2

Total CHO   neg
Total calories 320

Haddock with Courgettes

350g/12 oz haddock fillet
juice of 1 lemon
450g/1 lb courgettes, sliced
150ml/¼ pint fish stock (page 64)
1 × 2.5ml spoon/½ teaspoon dill seeds
1 × 2.5ml spoon/½ teaspoon fennel

1 × 2.5ml spoon/½ teaspoon parsley
salt, pepper

Garnish
2 × 15ml spoons/2 tablespoons
  canned sweetcorn

Divide the fish into two portions and put in a casserole.
Add the remaining ingredients and cook at
190°C/375°F/Gas 5 for 20 minutes. Garnish with the
sweetcorn.

Serving suggestion Whole new potatoes and runner beans

Serves 2

Total CHO   20g
Total calories 340

Hake with Cheese

1 lemon, sliced
225g/8 oz hake fillet
freshly ground black pepper
25g/1 oz Edam cheese, grated

Garnish
paprika

Put the lemon slices on the fish, sprinkle with pepper, and
wrap in foil. Put the parcel on a baking tray and cook at
180°C/350°F/Gas 4 for 20 minutes. Remove the lemon
slices, sprinkle with the cheese and place under a hot grill
until the cheese melts. Garnish with a sprinkling of paprika.

Serving suggestion Jacket potatoes and grilled tomatoes

Serves 2

Total CHO   neg
Total calories 250

Banana Trout

150ml/¼ pint fish stock (page 64)
2 × 15ml spoons/2 tablespoons dry
  white wine
1 medium onion, finely chopped
50g/2 oz fennel, chopped
juice of ½ lemon

white pepper
2 trout, ready gutted (150g/5 oz
  each)

Garnish
1 small banana, sliced

Put all the ingredients except the fish in a saucepan. Heat to boiling point, reduce the heat, cover and simmer for 15 minutes, add the fish and cook for a further 10 minutes. Drain, and place the trout on a serving dish. Garnish with slices of banana.

Serving suggestion Creamed potatoes and broccoli

Serves 2

Total CHO   20g
Total calories 300

Marinated Tuna

1 × 200g/7 oz can tuna in brine, drained
1 medium tomato, skinned and chopped
1 medium apple, cored and chopped
50g/2 oz button mushrooms, sliced
1 medium onion, finely chopped

2 × 15ml spoons/2 tablespoons wine
  vinegar
1 clove of garlic, crushed
1 × 2.5ml spoon/½ teaspoon dill seeds
juice of ½ lemon
salt, pepper

Mix all the ingredients together well and marinate for at least 2 hours before serving.

Serves 2
Total CHO   20g
Total calories 320

Serving suggestion Cold brown rice and any side salad

Casseroled Cod

675g/1½ lb cod fillet
3 medium onions, finely chopped
2 medium tomatoes, skinned and
  chopped
1 medium red pepper, deseeded and
  chopped
2 stalks celery, trimmed and chopped

juice of 1 lemon
2 × 15ml spoons/2 tablespoons
  Worcestershire sauce
3 × 15ml spoons/3 tablespoons cold
  water
1 bay leaf
fresh parsley
salt, pepper

Cut the fish into four pieces, and put into a casserole
with the other ingredients. Cook at 190°C/375°F/Gas 5 for
about 25 minutes.

Serves 4
Total CHO   20g
Total calories   620

Serving suggestion Jacket potatoes and spring greens

Salmon and Egg Mousse

2 × 15ml spoons/2 tablespoons water
3 × 5ml spoons/3 teaspoons gelatine
1 × 200g/7 oz can salmon, drained
3 size 3 eggs, hard-boiled and finely
  chopped
2 medium tomatoes, skinned and
  chopped
1 × 350g/12 oz can sweetcorn, drained

150g/5.3 oz natural yoghurt (1 small
  carton)
fresh parsley, chopped
1 × 5ml spoon/1 teaspoon celery salt
freshly ground black pepper

Garnish
cucumber slices

Put the water in a heatproof container, sprinkle in the
gelatine and leave to soften. Stand the container in a pan of
hot water and stir until the gelatine dissolves. Leave to cool,
then mix with the remaining ingredients. Pour into a 550ml/
1 pint mould and leave in a refrigerator until set. This will take
about 2 hours. Remove from the mould, and garnish with
cucumber slices.

Serves 4

Total CHO   60g
Total calories   900

Serving suggestion Whole new potatoes and any side salad

Baked Tuna with Broccoli

1 × 200g/7 oz can tuna in brine, drained
1 × 200g/7 oz can sweetcorn, drained
salt, pepper
225g/8 oz broccoli, broken into florets

150ml/¼ pint tomato juice
25g/1 oz Gouda cheese, grated
25g/1 oz fresh wholemeal breadcrumbs
1 × 5ml spoon/1 teaspoon oregano

Flake the tuna and put in an ovenproof dish. Cover with the sweetcorn, season and then cover with broccoli. Pour the tomato juice over the fish and vegetables. Mix together the cheese, breadcrumbs and oregano, and sprinkle on the fish to form a topping. Cook at 190°C/375°F/Gas 5 for about 25 minutes.

Serves 4

Total CHO   40g
Total calories 540

Serving suggestion Jacket potatoes and mixed vegetables

Crunchy Tuna Ring

2 × 15ml spoons/2 tablespoons water
3 × 5ml spoons/3 teaspoons gelatine
1 × 200g/7 oz can tuna in brine, drained
½ small cucumber, peeled and cubed
½ medium red pepper, deseeded and
 chopped
1 small onion, finely chopped
6 small gherkins, chopped
2 large tomatoes, skinned and chopped

1 × 15ml spoon/1 tablespoon
 low calorie salad cream
150g/5.3 oz natural yoghurt (1 small
 carton)
salt, pepper

Garnish
cucumber slices
tomato slices

Put the water in a heatproof container, sprinkle in the gelatine and leave to soften. Stand the container in a pan of hot water and stir until the gelatine dissolves. Leave to cool. Mix together the remaining ingredients and fold in the gelatine. Pour into a 550ml/1 pint ring mould and leave in a refrigerator until set. This will take about 2 hours. Remove from the ring mould and garnish with slices of cucumber and tomato.

Serves 4

Total CHO   20g
Total calories 400

Serving suggestion Whole new potatoes and sweetcorn

Stuffed Sole

50g/2 oz button mushrooms, sliced
4 stalks celery, trimmed and chopped
salt, pepper
juice of 1 lemon
4 small fillets of lemon sole (150g/
  5 oz each)

Garnish
tomato wedges
sprigs of parsley

Mix together the mushrooms, celery, salt, pepper and lemon juice. Place a quarter of the mixture in the centre of each fillet, roll up and secure with a cocktail stick. Place on a baking tray, cover with foil and cook at 180°C/350°F/Gas 4 for 20 minutes. Garnish with tomato wedges and sprigs of parsley.

Serves 4

Total CHO   *neg*
Total calories   *480*

Serving suggestion Whole new potatoes and runner beans

Shellfish

Prawns with Asparagus

100g/4 oz peeled prawns
100g/4 oz whole French beans
1 medium tomato, skinned and chopped
1 × 175g/6 oz can asparagus tips,
  drained

juice of ½ lemon
½ quantity of Yoghurt Dressing (1)
  (page 100)
lettuce
freshly ground black pepper

Mix together the prawns, beans, tomato, asparagus and lemon juice. Gently fold in the yoghurt dressing. Chill in a refrigerator and serve on a bed of crispy lettuce. Sprinkle with freshly ground black pepper.

Serves 2

Total CHO   *10g*
Total calories   *200*

Serving suggestion Whole new potatoes and sweetcorn

Pepper Prawns

1 × 5ml spoon / 1 teaspoon vegetable oil
1 medium onion, finely chopped
1 clove of garlic, crushed
1 medium green pepper, deseeded
  and chopped
225g / 8 oz peeled prawns
150ml / ¼ pint tomato juice

1 × 2.5ml spoon / ½ teaspoon celery salt
1 × 2.5ml spoon / ½ teaspoon fennel
1 × 2.5ml spoon / ½ teaspoon black
  pepper
4 × 15ml spoons / 4 tablespoons dry
  white wine
50g / 2 oz dried apricots, chopped

Heat the oil gently in a non-stick saucepan. Cook the onion, garlic and pepper for about 10 minutes until soft. Stir in the remaining ingredients, cover and simmer gently for a further 10 minutes. Sprinkle with freshly ground black pepper and serve immediately.

Serving suggestion Wholewheat pasta shells or noodles and whole green beans

Serves 2

Total CHO   **40g**
Total calories 480

Shrimps in Garlic Sauce

1 × 5ml spoon / 1 teaspoon vegetable oil
1 medium onion, finely chopped
3 cloves garlic, crushed
1 × 5ml spoon / 1 teaspoon
  concentrated tomato purée

6 × 15ml spoons / 6 tablespoons water
1 × 5ml spoon / 1 teaspoon oregano
freshly ground black pepper
350g / 12 oz peeled shrimps

Heat the oil in a non-stick frying pan and add the onion, garlic and tomato purée. Cook gently for 5 minutes and then add the water, oregano, black pepper and the shrimps. Cook gently for a further 10 minutes and serve immediately.

Serving suggestion Brown rice and whole French beans

Serves 4

Total CHO   **neg**
Total calories 480

Cold Seafood Medley

175g/6 oz peeled shrimps
1 × 200g/7 oz can tuna in brine, drained
175g/6 oz cod fillet, cooked and flaked
100g/4 oz button mushrooms, sliced
6 radishes, sliced
juice of 1 lemon

$\frac{1}{2}$ quantity of Yoghurt Dressing (1)
  (page 100)
salt, pepper

Garnish
paprika

Carefully mix together the shrimps, tuna and cod, the mushrooms, radishes and lemon juice. Fold in the yoghurt dressing and season to taste. Chill in a refrigerator and sprinkle with paprika before serving.

Serving suggestion Wholemeal baps and any side salad

Serves 4

Total CHO   **neg**
Total calories 500

Caribbean Prawns

225g/8 oz peeled prawns
1 medium red pepper, deseeded and
  chopped
1 × 275g/10 oz can mandarin oranges
  in natural juice
2 medium tomatoes, skinned and
  chopped
2 small bananas, sliced

1 small onion, finely chopped
1 small courgette, finely sliced
2 × 15ml spoons/2 tablespoons wine
  vinegar
salt, pepper
Chinese leaves

Garnish
cucumber slices

Mix together all the ingredients except the Chinese leaves and chill in a refrigerator. Serve on Chinese leaves, and garnish with slices of cucumber.

Serving suggestion Cold brown rice and any mixed salad

Serves 4
Total CHO   40g
Total calories 480

Crabmeat and Apple

1 × 200g/7 oz can crabmeat, drained
2 size 3 eggs, hard-boiled and chopped
450g/1 lb cooking apples, cored and
  sliced
½ small cucumber, cubed

2 medium onions, finely chopped
juice of 1 lemon
½ quantity of Tofu Dressing (page 99)
freshly ground black pepper

Mix together the crabmeat, eggs, apples, cucumber and
onions, then add the lemon juice and fold in the Tofu
dressing. Chill, and sprinkle with black pepper before serving.

Serves 4
Total CHO   60g
Total calories 680

Serving suggestion Cold brown rice and any side salad

Fish Stock

550ml/1 pint water
fish bones
1 × 5ml spoon/1 teaspoon tarragon
1 × 5ml spoon/1 teaspoon mixed dried
  herbs

1 clove of garlic
1 bay leaf
freshly ground black pepper
a slice of lemon

Put all the ingredients in a large saucepan, heat to boiling
point, reduce the heat, cover and simmer for 30 minutes. Pass
through a sieve and season to taste. Use as required.

Total CHO   neg
Total calories neg

Other Main Courses

It makes good economic and slimming sense to include a few dishes without meat in your weekly diet, and the recipes in the first section of this chapter show just how easy it is to prepare interesting and satisfying vegetable dishes.

The main-course salads which follow present new ways of approaching salads guaranteed to enliven any diet.

Baked Rice and Tomato

100g/4 oz brown rice
1 × 5ml spoon/1 teaspoon vegetable oil
1 medium onion, finely chopped
1 clove of garlic, crushed
275ml/½ pint water

1 × 5ml spoon/1 teaspoon oregano
1 × 5ml spoon/1 teaspoon basil
2 large tomatoes, chopped
salt, pepper
1 beef stock cube

Put the rice in a pan of boiling salted water and cook for about 25 minutes. Drain and rinse, then put in an ovenproof dish. Heat the oil in a saucepan and cook the onion and garlic gently for 5 minutes until soft. Add the water, herbs, tomato and seasoning, and crumble in the stock cube. Mix with the rice and cook at 180°C/350°F/Gas 4 for 25 minutes.

Serves 2

Total CHO **90g**
Total calories **480**

Serving suggestion Any pulse salad

Mushroom Pie

100g/4 oz mushrooms, sliced
1 × 5ml spoon/1 teaspoon mixed herbs
1 small onion, finely chopped
1 × 15ml spoon/1 tablespoon
  Worcestershire sauce

150ml/¼ pint tomato juice
50g/2 oz fresh wholemeal breadcrumbs
1 × 5ml spoon/1 teaspoon celery salt
freshly ground black pepper

Put the mushrooms, herbs and onion in an ovenproof dish. Pour over the Worcestershire sauce and tomato juice, and sprinkle with the breadcrumbs and celery salt. Season to taste, and cook at 180°C/350°F/Gas 4 for 25 minutes.

Serves 2

Total CHO **30g**
Total calories **180**

Serving suggestion Plain omelets and wholemeal rolls

Cabbage Cheese Bake

175g/6 oz white cabbage, shredded
2 medium tomatoes, skinned and sliced
150ml/¼ pint tomato juice
1 × 2.5ml spoon/½ teaspoon basil

1 × 2.5ml spoon/½ teaspoon oregano
salt, pepper
50g/2 oz Edam cheese, grated

Put the cabbage in an ovenproof dish and cover with the tomatoes, tomato juice and the mixed herbs. Season to taste, and then sprinkle with the grated cheese. Cover and cook at 180°C/350°F/Gas 4 for 25 minutes. Serve hot or cold.

Serving suggestion Any dried bean and rice salad

Serves 2

Total CHO   10g
Total calories 220

Cheese and Onion Crumble

1 small onion, finely chopped
50g/2 oz Edam cheese, grated
50g/2 oz fresh wholemeal breadcrumbs
150ml/¼ pint skimmed milk
salt, pepper

paprika

Garnish
tomato slices

Cover the base of an ovenproof dish with the onion. Mix together the cheese, breadcrumbs, skimmed milk, salt and pepper, and spread the mixture over the onions, Sprinkle with paprika. Cook at 230°C/450°F/Gas 8 for 10 minutes, then garnish with tomato slices, and serve immediately.

Serving suggestion Jacket potatoes and sweetcorn

Serves 2

Total CHO   30g
Total calories 320

Cheese Meringue

4 size 3 eggs, separated
4 × 15ml spoons/4 tablespoons natural
  yoghurt

25g/1 oz Edam cheese, grated
freshly ground black pepper

Whisk the egg whites until stiff and pour into an ovenproof
dish. Make four small dents in the whites and add the yolks.
Cover the yolks with the yoghurt, and sprinkle with the grated
cheese. Cook at 180°C/350°F/Gas 4 for 20 minutes, then
sprinkle with black pepper and serve immediately.

Serving suggestion Whole new potatoes and runner beans

Serves 2

Total CHO   *neg*
Total calories *400*

Cottage Fruit Savoury

100g/4 oz cottage cheese
150g/5.3 oz natural yoghurt (1 small
  carton)
1 large orange, chopped
1/2 small grapefruit, chopped
1/2 medium apple, cored and chopped

1/2 large pear, cored and chopped

Garnish
cucumber slices
paprika

Mix all the ingredients together well and chill in a refrigerator.
Garnish with cucumber slices and a sprinkling of paprika.

Serving suggestion Brown rice and any side salad

Serves 2
Total CHO   *30g*
Total calories *280*

Mushroom Bake

225g/8 oz button mushrooms, sliced
100g/4 oz cottage cheese
25g/1 oz Parmesan cheese, grated
2 medium onions, finely chopped
juice of 1/2 lemon

salt, pepper

Garnish
sprigs of parsley
lemon wedges

Put the mushrooms in an ovenproof dish. Mix together the
cottage cheese, Parmesan cheese, onions, lemon juice, salt
and pepper, then spread the mixture over the mushrooms.
Cook at 190°C/375°F/Gas 5 for 30 minutes. Garnish with
sprigs of parsley and lemon wedges, and serve immediately.

Serving Suggestion Jacket potatoes, and carrots and peas

Serves 2

Total CHO   *10g*
Total calories *260*

Parmesan Spinach Bake

675g/1½ lb spinach, chopped
1 medium onion, chopped
175g/6 oz mushrooms, sliced

1 × 5ml spoon/1 teaspoon oregano
salt, pepper
50g/2 oz Parmesan cheese, grated

Cook the spinach in a little boiling salted water for about 5 minutes until tender. Drain well. Transfer to an ovenproof dish with the onion, mushrooms, oregano, salt and pepper. Sprinkle the cheese over the top, and cook at 200°C/400°F/Gas 6 for 10 minutes until the cheese is bubbling. Serve immediately.

Serving suggestion Wholemeal rolls

Serves 4

Total CHO   20g
Total calories   360

Egg and Tomato Hats

2 large tomatoes
2 size 3 eggs, hard-boiled and chopped
fresh parsley, chopped
salt,pepper

lettuce

Garnish
sweetcorn

Cut the tops off the tomatoes and, using a teaspoon, remove the pulp. Mix the pulp with the egg, parsley, salt and pepper. Use the mixture to fill the tomato shells, then replace the tops. Serve on a bed of lettuce and garnish with sweetcorn.

Serving suggestion Any dried bean and pulse salad

Serves 2

Total CHO   neg
Total calories   180

Eggs Florentine

1 × 15ml spoon/1 tablespoon
  wholemeal/wholewheat flour
150g/5.3 oz natural yoghurt (1 small
  carton)
450g/1 lb spinach, chopped

freshly grated nutmeg
salt, pepper
2 size 3 eggs
25g/1 oz Parmesan cheese, grated

Mix the flour with a little cold water and fold into the yoghurt.
Put this mixture in a saucepan and heat gently to boiling point,
stirring all the time. Leave to cool.

Serves 2

Sprinkle the spinach with nutmeg and cook in boiling salted
water for about 5 minutes. Drain well, season to taste, and put
in a baking dish. Make two hollows in the spinach, and break
one egg into each. Pour the cooled yoghurt mixture over the
spinach and eggs, and sprinkle with cheese. Cook at
200°C/400°F/Gas 6 for 15 minutes until the eggs have set.

Total CHO   **30g**
Total calories **420**

Serving suggestion Whole new potatoes

Herb Omelet

3 size 3 eggs, separated
1 × 5ml spoon/1 teaspoon mixed herbs
2 × 15ml spoons/2 tablespoons water
salt, pepper

1 × 5ml spoon/1 teaspoon sunflower oil

Garnish
tomato slices

Beat together the egg yolks, mixed herbs, water, salt and
pepper. Whisk the egg whites until stiff and fold into the yolk
mixture. Heat the oil in an omelet pan and cook the egg
mixture until it just begins to set, then place under a hot grill
for 1 minute to seal the top. Garnish with tomato slices and
serve immediately.

Serves 2

Total CHO   **neg**
Total calories **280**

Serving suggestion Any green salad and wholemeal rolls

Cheese-topped Oat and Aubergine

50g/2 oz oatmeal
2 medium aubergines
1 × 5ml spoon/1 teaspoon vegetable oil
2 medium onions, finely chopped
175g/6 oz mushrooms, chopped

1 × 5ml spoon/1 teaspoon chervil
1 × 5ml spoon/1 teaspoon oregano
1 clove of garlic, crushed
salt, pepper
175g/6 oz Gruyère cheese, grated

Serves 4

Pour boiling water over the oatmeal and leave to stand overnight. Prick the skins of the aubergines with a fork, and bake at 190°C/375°F/Gas 5 for 20 minutes. Leave to cool, then scoop out the flesh. Gently heat the oil and sauté the onions and mushrooms until soft, then add the herbs, garlic, salt and pepper. Drain the oatmeal and mix with the vegetables. Pour into an ovenproof dish and cover with the cheese. Cook at 190°C/375°F/Gas 5 for 20 minutes.

Total CHO   60g
Total calories 900

Serving suggestion Any side salad

Cauliflower Cheese

1 large cauliflower, trimmed and cut into
  quarters
25g/1 oz low fat margarine
25g/1 oz wholemeal/wholewheat flour
550ml/1 pint skimmed milk

1 × 5ml spoon/1 teaspoon dry English
  mustard
1 × 5ml spoon/1 teaspoon celery salt
freshly ground black pepper
100g/4 oz Edam cheese, grated

Serves 4

Cook the cauliflower in boiling salted water for about 15 minutes. Melt the margarine in a saucepan and stir in the wholemeal flour. Cook for 3 minutes, stirring all the time. Remove from the heat and stir in the milk, mustard, celery salt and black pepper. Stir in the cheese and continue to stir until it melts. Pour over the cooked cauliflower and sprinkle with freshly ground black pepper.

Total CHO   60g
Total calories 760

Serving suggestion Whole french beans

Royal Mushrooms on Toast

1 × 5ml spoon/1 teaspoon sunflower oil
1 medium onion, chopped
225g/8 oz mushrooms, sliced
1 × 5ml spoon/1 teaspoon wholemeal/
  wholewheat flour
1 × 2.5ml spoon/½ teaspoon parsley
1 × 2.5ml spoon/½ teaspoon coriander

1 × 15ml spoon/1 tablespoon dry white
  wine
150g/5.3 oz natural yoghurt (1 small
  carton)
4 large slices wholemeal bread

Garnish
cress

Serves 4

Heat the oil in a saucepan and cook the onion and
mushrooms gently for 5 minutes. Mix the flour with a little cold
water, and stir into the onions and mushrooms. Cook for a
further 3 minutes, then add the herbs, wine and yoghurt. Toast
the bread, and cover each slice with the mushroom mixture.
Place under a grill for 3 minutes until bubbling, and garnish
with cress.

Total CHO	***80g***
Total calories	***560***

Serving suggestion Scrambled eggs

Slimmer's Hamburgers

75g/3 oz chick-peas
2 medium carrots, finely chopped
2 medium onions, finely chopped
1 medium green pepper, deseeded and
  finely chopped
2 stalks celery, trimmed and finely
  chopped

1 × 2.5ml spoon/½ teaspoon parsley
1 × 2.5ml spoon/½ teaspoon thyme
1 × 2.5ml spoon/½ teaspoon celery salt
freshly ground black pepper
2 size 3 eggs, well beaten

Serves 4

Soak the chick-peas in water overnight. Put in a saucepan
with sufficient salted water, and heat to boiling point. Reduce
the heat, cover and simmer for 1 hour. Alternatively, cook the
chick-peas, in a pressure cooker.

Steam the vegetables, with the herbs and seasoning for
about 15 minutes until tender.

Mash the chick-peas, and mix together with the vegetables
and the beaten egg. Form into four small patties, and grill on
either side for 10 minutes.

Total CHO	***60g***
Total calories	***360***

Serving suggestion Wholemeal baps and any side salad

Spinach and Cheese Pie

675g/1½ lb fresh spinach, chopped **or**
  450g/1 lb frozen spinach, thawed and
  chopped
175g/6 oz cottage cheese
salt, pepper
1 × 5ml spoon/1 teaspoon oregano
450g/1 lb tomatoes, skinned and sliced

100g/4 oz Cheddar cheese, grated
25g/1 oz Parmesan cheese, grated
25g/1 oz wholemeal breadcrumbs

Garnish
tomato slices
sprigs of parsley

Cook the fresh spinach in boiling salted water for about 10 minutes until tender. Drain well. Mix the steamed spinach or the frozen spinach together with the cottage cheese, salt, pepper and oregano. Put the mixture in an ovenproof dish and cover with alternate layers of sliced tomato and Cheddar cheese. Cover with a mixture of the Parmesan cheese and breadcrumbs. Bake at 200°C/400°F/Gas 6 for 15 minutes, or until bubbling. Garnish with tomato slices and sprigs of parsley.

Serves 4

Total CHO   ***40g***
Total calories ***860***

Serving suggestion Jacket potatoes and sweetcorn

Spicy Cabbage

1 × 5ml spoon/1 teaspoon soya bean
  oil
1 large onion, finely chopped
450g/1 lb white cabbage, finely
  shredded
5 × 15ml spoons/5 tablespoons dry
  white wine
2 × 5ml spoons/2 teaspoons made
  French mustard
1 × 5ml spoon/1 teaspoon curry powder

2 × 15ml spoons/2 tablespoons sultanas
1 × 5ml spoon/1 teaspoon celery salt
freshly ground black pepper
2 size 3 eggs, well beaten
100g/4 oz cooked brown rice

Garnish
tomato wedges
fresh parsley, chopped

Heat the oil in a large non-stick saucepan. Add the onion and cabbage, and cook gently for 5 minutes, stirring all the time.

   Mix together the rest of the ingredients and add to the vegetables. Cook gently for a further 5 minutes. Garnish with tomato wedges and chopped parsley, and serve with soy sauce.

Serves 4

Total CHO   ***60g***
Total calories ***580***

Serving suggestion Jacket potatoes and broad beans

Mozzarella Casserole

1 × 400g/14 oz can tomatoes
2 small cucumbers, peeled and cubed
1 medium green pepper, deseeded and
  chopped
3 medium onions, chopped
2 cloves garlic, crushed
salt, pepper
150ml/¼ pint water

1 chicken stock cube
25g/1 oz Parmesan cheese, grated
1 × 5ml spoon/1 teaspoon oregano
225g/8 oz Mozzarella cheese, grated

Garnish
tomato slices

Put all the vegetables in an ovenproof dish with the garlic, salt
and pepper. Add the water, and crumble in the stock cube.
Sprinkle with the Parmesan cheese, oregano and Mozzarella
cheese. Cook at 190°C/375°F/Gas 5 for 20 minutes.
Garnish with tomato slices and serve immediately.

Serving suggestion Brown rice and broccoli

Serves 4

Total CHO   **10g**
Total calories   **880**

Main-Course Salads

Adukie Bean Salad

100g/4 oz adukie beans
juice of ½ lemon
1 medium onion, chopped
1 medium red pepper, deseeded and
  chopped

2 cloves garlic, crushed
salt, pepper
½ quantity of Vinaigrette (page 99)

Soak the beans in water overnight, drain off the water and
rinse well. Put them in a saucepan with sufficient salted water,
and add the lemon juice. Heat to boiling point, reduce the
heat, cover and simmer for 1 hour. Alternatively, cook the
beans in a pressure cooker. Rinse the cooked beans in cold
water, drain, and leave to cool. Mix with the other ingredients,
and leave to stand for at least 2 hours before serving.

Serving suggestion Cottage cheese

Serves 2

Total CHO   **40g**
Total calories   **280**

Cottage Cheese and Melon Salad

½ small honeydew melon, skinned, deseeded and cubed
1 medium red-skinned apple, cored and sliced
1 medium green-skinned apple, cored and sliced

150g/5 oz cottage cheese
juice of ½ lemon
paprika
lettuce

Mix the fruit together and carefully fold in the cottage cheese and lemon juice. Season to taste with paprika, and chill in a refrigerator. Serve on a bed of lettuce.

Serves 2
Total CHO   40g
Total calories 300

Garlic Chicken Salad

175g/6 oz cooked chicken, diced
½ quantity of Vinaigrette (page 99)
1 medium apple, cored and sliced
1 medium onion, finely chopped

2 cloves garlic, crushed
salt, pepper
fresh beansprouts

Put the chicken in the vinaigrette dressing and marinate for 2 hours. Add the remaining ingredients, and mix well. Serve on a bed of fresh beansprouts.

Serves 2
Total CHO   10g
Total calories 320

Tuna Fish Salad

1 × 200g/7 oz can tuna in brine, drained
1 small onion, chopped
2 medium tomatoes, skinned and
   chopped
2 stalks celery, trimmed and chopped
1 medium green pepper, deseeded and
   chopped

½ small cucumber, peeled and cubed
3 × 15ml spoons/3 tablespoons tomato
   juice
1 × 5ml spoon/1 teaspoon basil
salt, pepper
Chinese leaves, chopped **or** lettuce,
   shredded

Flake the tuna and mix with all the remaining ingredients,
except the leaves or lettuce. Serve with the leaves or lettuce.

Serves 4
Total CHO   10g
Total calories 280

Prawn Salad

350g/12 oz peeled prawns
1 medium red pepper, deseeded and
   chopped
2 medium tomatoes, skinned and
   chopped
4 stalks celery, trimmed and chopped
2 × 15ml spoons/2 tablespoons wine
   vinegar

juice of 1 lemon
150g/5.3 oz natural yoghurt (1 small
   carton)
salt, pepper

Garnish
sprigs of watercress
lemon twists

Put the prawns and vegetables into a bowl. Mix together the
vinegar, lemon juice, yoghurt and seasoning, and use to toss
the salad. Garnish with watercress and lemon twists.

Serves 4
Total CHO   10g
Total calories 420

Prawn and Avocado Salad

225g/8 oz peeled prawns
1 medium avocado pear, stoned and
  sliced
225g/8 oz button mushrooms
2 medium tomatoes, sliced
1 medium red pepper, deseeded and
  sliced

1 × 2.5ml spoon/½ teaspoon mint
1 × 2.5ml spoon/½ teaspoon celery salt
freshly ground black pepper

Garnish
sprigs of watercress

Put the prawns, avocado and vegetables into a bowl. Add the
seasoning and mix well. Garnish with sprigs of watercress.

Serves 4
Total CHO   10g
Total calories   640

Shrimp and Walnut Salad

350g/12 oz peeled shrimps
2 medium eating apples, cored and
  sliced
50g/2 oz shelled walnuts, chopped
juice of 1 lemon
150g/5.3 oz natural yoghurt (1 small
  carton)

salt, pepper
lettuce, chopped

Garnish
paprika

Mix together the shrimps, apples, walnuts and lemon juice.
Fold in the yoghurt and seasoning, and serve on a bed of
chopped lettuce. Chill in a refrigerator and sprinkle with
paprika before serving.

Serves 4

Total CHO   40g
Total calories   860

Cottage Salad

450g/1 lb white cabbage, finely
  shredded
450g/1 lb courgettes, sliced
1 medium orange, chopped
1 bulb of fennel, trimmed and chopped
225g/8 oz cottage cheese

½ quantity of Yoghurt Dressing (1)
  (page 100)
salt, pepper

Garnish
mustard and cress

Mix all the ingredients together well and chill in a refrigerator
before serving. Garnish with mustard and cress.

Serves 4
Total CHO   40g
Total calories   460

American Club Salad

100g/4 oz cooked chicken, chopped
100g/4 oz lean cooked ham, chopped
100g/4 oz cooked tongue, chopped
1 × 225g/8 oz can bamboo shoots,
  drained
1 lettuce
1 small cucumber, peeled and cubed
1 medium green pepper, deseeded and
  chopped

1 clove of garlic, crushed
½ quantity of Vinaigrette (page 99)
salt, pepper

Garnish
thin tomato slices
fresh parsley, chopped

Put all the ingredients in a large salad bowl and mix together
well. Garnish with thin slices of tomato and chopped parsley.

Serves 4
Total CHO   10g
Total calories 600

Frankfurter and Rice Salad

75g/3 oz brown rice
1 × 275g/10 oz can frankfurters, drained
½ medium red pepper, deseeded and
  chopped
½ medium green pepper, deseeded and
  chopped

fresh parsley, chopped
1 × 5ml spoon/1 teaspoon celery salt
freshly ground black pepper

Garnish
sprigs of parsley
tomato wedges

Put the rice in a saucepan of boiling salted water and cook for
about 45 minutes. Drain and rinse, then leave to cool. Slice the
frankfurters finely and mix together with the rice and the
remaining ingredients. Garnish with sprigs of parsley and
tomato wedges.

Serves 4

Total CHO   80g
Total calories 820

Shredded Wheat Salad

4 shredded wheat biscuits
150g/5.3 oz natural yoghurt (1 small
  carton)
100g/4 oz cottage cheese
1 × 200g/7 oz can sweetcorn, drained
2 stalks celery, trimmed and chopped

3 × 15ml spoons/3 tablespoons wine
  vinegar
salt, pepper

Garnish
cucumber slices
tomato slices

Break up the biscuits and put in a salad bowl with the other
ingredients. Mix together well. Chill in a refrigerator and
garnish with slices of cucumber and tomato.

Serves 4

Total CHO   100g
Total calories   660

Oatmeal Salad

50g/2 oz coarse oatmeal
225g/8 oz cottage cheese
1 small onion, sliced
1 medium apple, cored and sliced
1 medium red pepper, deseeded and
  chopped

25g/1 oz fresh parsley, chopped
salt, freshly ground black pepper
ground nutmeg
cress

Pour boiling water over the oatmeal and leave to stand
overnight. Mix together all the remaining ingredients, except
the cress, add to the oatmeal, and mix well. Chill in a
refrigerator, and serve on a bed of cress.

Serves 4

Total CHO   60g
Total calories 480

Sunflower Rice Salad

50g/2 oz brown rice
1 × 5ml spoon/1 teaspoon turmeric
25g/1 oz sunflower seeds
2 medium onions, chopped
1/2 medium red pepper, deseeded and
  chopped

1/2 fresh chilli, deseeded and chopped
1 clove of garlic, crushed
fresh parsley, chopped
salt, pepper
1/2 quantity of Vinaigrette (page 99)

Put the rice and turmeric in a saucepan of boiling salted water and cook for about 45 minutes. Drain and rinse the rice. Leave to cool, then mix together with the sunflower seeds, onions, pepper, chilli, garlic, parsley and seasoning. Pour over the vinaigrette dressing. Leave to stand for 2 hours before serving.

Serves 4

Total CHO **60g**
Total calories **400**

Wholewheat Pasta Salad

100g/4 oz wholewheat pasta, eg shells
  or macaroni
2 medium carrots, sliced
1 medium green pepper, deseeded and
  chopped
4 stalks celery, trimmed and chopped

1 × 2.5ml spoon/1/2 teaspoon garlic
  powder
1 × 15ml spoon/1 tablespoon
  Worcestershire sauce

Garnish
fresh parsley, chopped

Put the pasta in a pan of boiling salted water and cook for 15-20 minutes. Drain, and leave until cool. Mix with the remaining ingredients, and garnish with chopped parsley.

Serves 4
Total CHO **80g**
Total calories **400**

Vegetables and Side Salads

Cooked vegetables or side salads add bulk, fibre, vitamins and minerals to your diet, but very few calories. They are, therefore, important accompaniments to your main course dish.

Vegetables

Courgettes with Herbs

450g/1 lb courgettes, sliced
2 medium onions, finely chopped
150ml/$\frac{1}{4}$ pint tomato juice
1 × 2.5ml spoon/$\frac{1}{2}$ teaspoon basil
sprigs of parsley

salt, pepper

Garnish
fresh mint, chopped

Put the courgettes and onions in a large saucepan. Add the tomato juice, basil, parsley and seasoning. Heat slowly to boiling point, reduce the heat, cover and simmer for 15 minutes. Season to taste, and garnish with chopped mint. Serve hot or cold.

Serves 2

Total CHO   **30g**
Total calories   **300**

Festive Mushrooms

3 × 15ml spoons/3 tablespoons white
  wine vinegar
2 cloves
2 sticks cinnamon
225g/8 oz button mushrooms, sliced

150g/5.3 oz natural yoghurt (1 small
  carton)

Garnish
red pepper, chopped

Put the vinegar, cloves and cinnamon sticks in a saucepan. Heat to boiling point, reduce the heat, cover and simmer for 5 minutes. Add the mushrooms to the liquid and simmer for a further 10 minutes, with the lid off the pan, until the liquid has evaporated. Place on a serving dish, cover with the yoghurt and garnish with chopped red pepper.

Serves 2

Total CHO   **10g**
Total calories   **110**

Marrow Casserole

1 small marrow, deseeded and sliced
1 medium red pepper, deseeded and
  sliced
2 medium courgettes, sliced
2 medium tomatoes, sliced

2 cloves garlic, crushed
150ml/¼ pint tomato juice
1 × 5ml spoon/1 teaspoon basil
1 × 5ml spoon/1 teaspoon oregano
salt, pepper

Put all the ingredients in a large casserole. Cook at
190°C/375°F/Gas 5 for 45 minutes. Serve hot.

Serves 2
Total CHO   30g
Total calories   160

Serving suggestion Jacket potatoes and any lean oven-
baked chop

Vegetable Compôte

225g/8 oz courgettes, sliced
350g/12 oz cauliflower, broken into
  florets
2 medium onions, chopped
1 small green pepper, deseeded and
  chopped
1 small red pepper, deseeded and
  chopped

75g/3 oz frozen peas
150ml/¼ pint cold water
juice of 1 lemon
1 × 5ml spoon/1 teaspoon celery salt
freshly ground black pepper
1 chicken stock cube

Put all the vegetables in a large saucepan. Add the water,
lemon juice and seasoning, and crumble in the stock cube.
Heat to boiling point, reduce the heat, cover and simmer for
20 minutes.

Serves 4

Total CHO   20g
Total calories   180

Serving suggestion Roast chicken or sliced meat

Bouquet of Vegetables

100g/4 oz green peas, cooked
100g/4 oz whole runner beans, cooked
100g/4 oz mushrooms, sliced
½ small cucumber, cubed
1 large onion, chopped
100g/4 oz radishes, sliced
100g/4 oz cauliflower, broken into florets

1 medium red pepper, deseeded and
  chopped
1 × 5ml spoon/1 teaspoon celery salt
1 clove of garlic, crushed
freshly ground black pepper
150ml/¼ pint tomato juice

Mix all the vegetables and seasoning together in a large salad bowl. Pour in the tomato juice, and marinate for 12 hours before serving.

Serving suggestion Any cold meat

Serves 4
Total CHO   20g
Total calories   200

Harlequin Vegetables

1 medium aubergine, skinned and thinly
  sliced
450g/1 lb courgettes, sliced
1 medium red pepper, deseeded and
  sliced
1 medium green pepper, deseeded and
  sliced
2 medium tomatoes, skinned and
  chopped
275ml/½ pint tomato juice

2 × 5ml spoons/2 teaspoons curry
  powder
2 cloves garlic, crushed
2 × 15ml spoons/2 tablespoons
  Worcestershire sauce
salt, pepper

Garnish
tomato slices
fresh parsley, chopped

Put all the ingredients in a large saucepan. Heat to boiling point, reduce the heat, cover and simmer for 30 minutes. Turn the cooked vegetables into a glass serving bowl and leave to cool. Garnish with slices of tomato and chopped parsley.

Serves 4

Total CHO   30g
Total calories   150

Caraway Cabbage

450g/1 lb white cabbage, finely
  shredded
450g/1 lb cooking apples, peeled, cored
  and sliced

juice of 1 lemon
1 × 5ml spoon/1 teaspoon caraway
  seeds
2 × 15ml spoons/2 tablespoons currants
  or raisins

Mix the cabbage and apple together in a large salad bowl.
Add the lemon juice, caraway seeds and dried fruit, and leave
to stand for at least 2 hours before serving.

Serves 4
Total CHO   **60g**
Total calories **260**

Slavic Cabbage

675g/1½ lb white cabbage, shredded
2 medium onions, finely chopped
juice of 1 lemon
1 × 15ml spoon/1 tablespoon sunflower
  oil
1 × 15ml spoon/1 tablespoon wine
  vinegar

1 × 5ml spoon/1 teaspoon celery salt
freshly ground black pepper

Garnish
2 size 3 eggs, hard-boiled and chopped
parsley

Mix the cabbage and onions together in a salad bowl. Make a
dressing by mixing together the lemon juice, oil, vinegar,
celery salt and black pepper, and pour this over the
vegetables. Combine the egg and parsley, and sprinkle over
the top. Chill in a refrigerator.

Serves 4

Total CHO   **40g**
Total calories **500**

Serving suggestion Cold meats

Pickled Cabbage

450g/1 lb red cabbage, finely shredded
50g/2 oz salt
550ml/1 pint red wine vinegar
2 cloves
2 cloves garlic, crushed

1 × 2.5ml spoon/½ teaspoon nutmeg
1 × 2.5ml spoon/½ teaspoon black
  peppercorns
1 × 2.5ml spoon/½ teaspoon dried,
  chopped chillies

Lay the cabbage on a flat plate and sprinkle with the salt.
Leave for 24 hours, then refresh in cold water. Rinse well.
Pack the cabbage into sterilized screw-topped jars. Mix the
vinegar with the herbs and spices and pour over the cabbage.
Put on vinegar-proof covers, and seal the jars tightly.
Note This cabbage will keep well for up to a month if stored in
a cool dry place.

Serves 4

Total CHO   **15g**
Total calories   **90**

Horseradish Cauliflower

1 large cauliflower, broken into florets
4 × 15ml spoons/4 tablespoons bottled
  grated horseradish
150ml/¼ pint cold water
25g/1 oz fresh parsley, chopped
1 × 5ml spoon/1 teaspoon celery salt

freshly ground black pepper
150g/5.3 oz natural yoghurt (1 small
  carton)

Garnish
fresh parsley, chopped

Put the cauliflower in a large saucepan with the grated
horseradish, water, parsley, celery salt and black pepper.
Heat to boiling point, reduce the heat, cover and simmer for
15 minutes. Place in a serving dish, pour over the yoghurt,
and sprinkle with chopped parsley.

Serves 4

Total CHO   **20g**
Total calories **140**

German Red Cabbage

450g/1 lb red cabbage, finely shredded
450g/1 lb cooking apples, cored and
  chopped

275ml/½ pint cold water
3 × 15ml spoons/3 tablespoons wine
  vinegar
salt, pepper

Put the cabbage and apples in a large saucepan, and add the water, vinegar and seasoning. Heat to boiling point, reduce the heat, cover and simmer for 20 minutes. Drain well, and serve hot or cold.

Serving suggestion Sliced lean meats

Serves 4

Total CHO **40g**
Total calories **200**

Side Salads

Curried Rice Salad

50g/2 oz brown rice, cooked
2 medium onions, chopped
2 cloves garlic, crushed

2 × 5ml spoons/2 teaspoons curry
  powder
1 × 5ml spoon/1 teaspoon cinnamon
salt, pepper

Put the rice and onions into a bowl. Add the garlic and spices, mix well together and season to taste.

Serving suggestion Cold meats or sliced hard-boiled eggs

Serves 2
Total CHO **50g**
Total calories **250**

Chinese Leaf Salad

175g/6 oz Chinese leaves, chopped
1 medium onion, chopped
1 medium apple, cored and sliced
1 medium tomato, skinned and chopped
½ medium green pepper, deseeded and
  chopped

½ medium red pepper, deseeded and
  chopped
1 × 2.5ml spoon/½ teaspoon chervil
1 × 2.5ml spoon/½ teaspoon celery salt
freshly ground black pepper

Put the vegetables and fruit in a salad bowl, add the herbs and seasoning, and mix well together.

Serves 2
Total CHO **20g**
Total calories **110**

Beansprout and Radish Salad

150g/5 oz beansprouts
1 medium pepper, deseeded and
  sliced
4 stalks celery, trimmed and sliced
50g/2 oz radishes, sliced

1 clove of garlic, crushed
4 × 15ml spoons/4 tablespoons wine
  vinegar
1 × 15ml spoon/1 tablespoon soy
  sauce
salt, pepper

Put the vegetables into a salad bowl, and add the garlic, vinegar, soy sauce and seasoning. Mix together well, and leave to stand for at least 2 hours before serving.

Serves 2
Total CHO   neg
Total calories   40

Sweetcorn and Watercress Salad

1 bunch of watercress
1 × 200g/7 oz can sweetcorn, drained
2 medium tomatoes, skinned and
  chopped
1 × 15ml spoon/1 tablespoon wine
  vinegar

1 × 5ml spoon/1 teaspoon celery salt
freshly ground black pepper

Garnish
cucumber slices

Mix together the watercress, sweetcorn, tomatoes and vinegar in a salad bowl. Season to taste, and garnish with cucumber slices.

Serves 2
Total CHO   20g
Total calories   100

Cucumber and Sweetcorn Salad

1 medium red pepper, deseeded and
 chopped
1 medium onion, chopped
1 × 200g/7 oz can sweetcorn, drained
1 small cucumber, peeled and cubed
150g/5.3 oz natural yoghurt (1 small
 carton)

juice of 1 lemon
1 × 15ml spoon/1 tablespoon wine
 vinegar
salt, freshly ground black pepper

Garnish
sprigs of watercress

Put the vegetables in a large salad bowl. Pour on the yoghurt,
lemon juice and vinegar, and season to taste. Mix together
well. Chill in a refrigerator and garnish with the watercress.

Serves 4
Total CHO   ***40g***
Total calories ***240***

Cucumber and Celery Crunch

1 medium cucumber, cubed
2 medium onions, finely chopped
1 medium green pepper, deseeded
 and chopped
4 stalks celery, trimmed and chopped
juice of 1 lemon

1 × 15ml spoon/1 tablespoon wine
 vinegar
1 × 5ml spoon/1 teaspoon celery salt
1 × 5ml spoon/1 teaspoon mixed herbs
freshly ground black pepper

Put the vegetables in a salad bowl, and add the lemon juice,
vinegar, celery salt, herbs and pepper. Mix well together, and
chill in a refrigerator before serving.

Serves 4
Total CHO   ***20g***
Total calories ***120***

Minty Leek Salad

½ small cucumber, peeled and cubed
½ small cabbage, finely shredded
2 medium leeks, trimmed and sliced
1 medium green pepper, deseeded and
  chopped
2 medium tomatoes, deseeded and
  chopped
1 medium onion, chopped

1 × 15ml spoon/1 tablespoon
  Worcestershire sauce
2 × 15ml spoons/2 tablespoons wine
  vinegar
fresh mint
2 cloves garlic, crushed
1 × 2.5ml spoon/½ teaspoon celery salt
freshly ground black pepper

Put the vegetables in a large salad bowl, add the
Worcestershire sauce, vinegar, herbs, garlic and seasoning,
and mix together well. Marinate for at least 2 hours before
serving.

Serves 4

Total CHO   20g
Total calories 160

Marinated Apple and Vegetable Salad

2 medium apples, cored and sliced
juice of 1 lemon
4 stalks celery, trimmed and chopped
225g/8 oz white cabbage, finely
  shredded
2 medium tomatoes, chopped

1 × 5ml spoon/1 teaspoon celery salt
freshly ground black pepper
½ quantity of Vinaigrette (page 99)

Garnish
caraway seeds

Put the apples in a bowl and cover with the lemon juice. Add
the celery, cabbage, tomatoes, celery salt and pepper. Pour
over the vinaigrette dressing and marinate in a refrigerator for
2 hours before serving. Garnish with caraway seeds.

Serves 4

Total CHO   30g
Total calories 160

Celery and Cottage Cheese Salad

4 stalks celery, trimmed and chopped
1 large apple, cored and sliced
1 medium onion, finely chopped
175g/6 oz cottage cheese
1 × 5ml spoon/1 teaspoon celery salt

freshly ground black pepper

Garnish
fresh chives, chopped

Put all the ingredients in a large salad bowl. Mix well together, and garnish with chopped chives.

Serves 4
Total CHO   20g
Total calories 240

Chinese Leaf and Pepper Salad

225g/8 oz Chinese leaves, chopped
1 medium onion, chopped
1 medium green pepper, deseeded and
  chopped

6 radishes, sliced
1 × 2.5ml spoon/½ teaspoon celery salt
freshly ground black pepper
½ quantity of Vinaigrette (page 99)

Put the vegetables in a large salad bowl. Add the seasoning, and pour on the vinaigrette dressing. Marinate for 2 hours before serving.

Serves 4
Total CHO   10g
Total calories   60

Crispy Chicory Salad

2 large oranges, chopped
225g/8 oz cottage cheese
fresh parsley, chopped
salt, pepper

½ quantity of Vinaigrette (page 99)
350g/12 oz chicory, chopped
Cayenne pepper

Mix together the orange pieces, cottage cheese, parsley, salt, pepper and vinaigrette dressing. Put the chicory on to a serving dish, make a well in the centre, and fill with the cottage cheese mixture. Chill in a refrigerator and sprinkle with Cayenne pepper before serving.

Serves 4

Total CHO   30g
Total calories 340

Coleslaw

450g/1 lb white cabbage, finely
  shredded
2 medium carrots, finely shredded
1 medium onion, finely chopped
salt, pepper

juice of 1 orange
5 × 15ml spoons/5 tablespoons wine
  vinegar
½ quantity of Mock Mayonnaise (page
  100)

Mix together the cabbage, carrots, onion, salt and pepper in a
large salad bowl. Mix together the orange juice and vinegar,
and pour over the vegetables. Marinate for 2 hours. Drain off
any excess liquid and fold in the mock mayonnaise. Serve
immediately.

Serves 4

Total CHO   40g
Total calories 280

Red Cabbage Salad

225g/8 oz red cabbage, shredded
2 stalks celery, trimmed and chopped
1 large cooking apple, cored and sliced
juice of ½ lemon
1 × 2.5ml spoon/½ teaspoon celery salt

freshly ground black pepper

Garnish
fresh parsley, chopped

Mix all the ingredients together well in a large salad bowl and
garnish with chopped parsley.

Serves 4
Total CHO   20g
Total calories 100

Bean Curd Salad

1 × 5ml spoon/1 teaspoon sunflower oil
1 medium onion, finely chopped
175g/6 oz beansprouts
1 piece of fresh root ginger
2 cloves garlic, crushed

1 chilli, deseeded and chopped
225g/8 oz soya bean curd (tofu)
5 × 15ml spoons/5 tablespoons dry
  white wine
salt, pepper

Heat the oil in a large non-stick saucepan. Add the onion,
beansprouts, ginger, garlic and chilli, and cook on medium
heat for 5 minutes, stirring all the time. Stir in the bean curd
and the wine, reduce the heat, and simmer gently for a further
5 minutes. Remove the ginger. Season to taste, and serve
immediately with a dash of soy sauce.

Serves 4

Total CHO   10g
Total calories 300

Beansprout Salad

175g/6 oz beansprouts
1 × 200g/7 oz can sweetcorn, drained
4 stalks celery, trimmed and chopped
175g/6 oz button mushrooms
50g/2 oz lentils, cooked
juice of 1 lemon

1 × 15ml spoon/1 tablespoon wine
  vinegar
salt, black pepper

Garnish
fresh mint

Mix all the ingredients together in a large salad bowl. Chill in a refrigerator, and garnish with fresh mint.

Serves 4
Total CHO   60g
Total calories 360

Oriental Salad

175g/6 oz beansprouts, chopped
175g/6 oz white cabbage, finely
  shredded
2 stalks celery, trimmed and chopped
3 medium onions, chopped
25g/1 oz almonds, chopped

1 small cooking apple, skinned, cored
  and sliced
1 × 15ml spoon/1 tablespoon soy sauce
salt, pepper
½ quantity of Vinaigrette (page 99)

Mix together in a large bowl the vegetables, nuts and the apple. Add the soy sauce, and season to taste. Pour over the vinaigrette dressing and marinate in a refrigerator for at least 2 hours.

Serves 4

Total CHO   40g
Total calories 340

Serving suggestion Brown rice and pineapple

Garden Salad

juice of 1 lemon
3 × 15ml spoons / 3 tablespoons wine
  vinegar
150ml / ¼ pint cold water
salt, pepper
3 × 5ml spoons / 3 teaspoons gelatine
1 medium carrot, grated
1 medium red-skinned apple, cored and
  grated

1 medium onion, chopped
2 medium tomatoes, chopped
2 stalks celery, trimmed and chopped

Garnish
radish roses
sprigs of watercress

Mix together in a heatproof container the lemon juice, vinegar, water, seasoning and gelatine. Leave until the gelatine softens, then stand the container in a pan of hot water and stir until the gelatine dissolves. Fill a glass bowl with separate layers of carrot, apple, onion, tomatoes and celery. Pour over the gelatine mixture and leave in a refrigerator until set. Turn out of the dish and garnish with radish roses and sprigs of watercress.

Serves 4

Total CHO   **20g**
Total calories **120**

Fruit and Vegetable Salad

½ small marrow, peeled and sliced
1 medium apple, cored and sliced
2 stalks celery, trimmed and chopped
2 medium tomatoes, chopped

1 × 5ml spoon / 1 teaspoon celery seeds
salt, black pepper
¼ quantity of Slim Salad Sauce (page
  104)

Mix together the marrow, apple, celery, tomatoes and celery seeds in a large salad bowl. Season to taste, and pour over the salad dressing. Marinate in a refrigerator for 2 hours before serving.

Serves 4

Total CHO   **20g**
Total calories **100**

Swisslaw

1 large apple, cored and sliced
1 stalk celery, trimmed and chopped
1 medium red pepper, deseeded and
  chopped
1 medium onion, chopped
1 large carrot, grated
50g/2 oz white cabbage, finely shredded
50g/2 oz red cabbage, finely shredded
fresh parsley, chopped
juice of 1 lemon
1 × 15ml spoon/1 tablespoon wine
  vinegar

1 × 2.5ml spoon/$\frac{1}{2}$ teaspoon oregano
1 × 2.5ml spoon/$\frac{1}{2}$ teaspoon curry
  powder
1 × 2.5ml spoon/$\frac{1}{2}$ teaspoon made
  English mustard
salt, pepper
150g/5.3 oz natural yoghurt (1 small
  carton)

Garnish
tomato wedges

Mix together the apple and vegetables in a large salad bowl.
Stir the lemon juice, vinegar, oregano, curry powder, mustard
and salt and pepper into the yoghurt and fold into the salad.
Chill in a refrigerator and garnish with tomato wedges.

Serves 4

Total CHO   40g
Total calories 220

Water Chestnut Salad

1 × 275g/10 oz can water chestnuts,
  drained and sliced
225g/8 oz beansprouts, chopped
1 medium onion, finely chopped
1 medium red pepper, deseeded and
  chopped

2 medium tomatoes, chopped
2 × 15ml spoons/2 tablespoons lemon
  juice
1 × 15ml spoon/1 tablespoon soy sauce
2 cloves garlic, crushed
salt, pepper
$\frac{1}{2}$ quantity of Vinaigrette (page 99)

Put the water chestnuts and vegetables in a large salad bowl,
add the lemon juice, soy sauce, garlic and seasoning. Mix
well together. Pour on the vinaigrette dressing and marinate
for 2 hours before serving.

Serves 4

Total CHO   40g
Total calories 180

Chutneys, Dressings and Sauces

These recipes are designed to help you add exciting flavours to your food, without adding extra calories. Chutneys, dressings and sauces enliven the taste-buds and enrich many recipes. Each one given here will keep well in a refrigerator for several days, so can be prepared ahead and used with a variety of dishes.

Chutneys

Banana Chutney

1 medium apple, peeled and cored
1 medium onion, chopped
2 small bananas, mashed
3 × 15ml spoons / 3 tablespoons spiced
  vinegar (page 95)

1 × 5ml spoon / 1 teaspoon nutmeg
1 × 5ml spoon / 1 teaspoon ground
  ginger
25g / 1 oz fructose
150ml / $\frac{1}{4}$ pint water

Put all the ingredients in a large saucepan. Heat to boiling point, reduce the heat, cover and simmer for 30 minutes. Leave to cool, then process in a blender until smooth. When cold, pour into a sterilized screw-topped jar and seal well. Serve with hard-boiled eggs, brown rice or cottage cheese.

Total CHO   *35g*
Total calories   *240*

Green Tomato Chutney

900g / 2 lb green tomatoes, chopped
2 large onions, chopped
50g / 2 oz fresh root ginger, chopped
50g / 2 oz sultanas

50g / 2 oz fructose
150ml / $\frac{1}{4}$ pint spiced vinegar (page 95)
salt, pepper

Put all the ingredients in a large saucepan. Heat to boiling point, reduce the heat, cover and simmer for 1 hour. Pour into sterilized screw-topped jars and seal well. Serve with cold meats, flans or on open sandwiches.

Total CHO   *80g*
Total calories   *550*

Marrow and Apple Chutney

1.8kg/4 lb cooking apples, cored and
  chopped
3 large onions, chopped
1 medium marrow, peeled and chopped

550ml/1 pint spiced vinegar
2 × 5ml spoons/2 teaspoons ground
  ginger
liquid sweetener

Put all the ingredients in a large saucepan. Heat to boiling
point, reduce the heat, cover and simmer for 1 hour, stirring
from time to time. Pour into sterilized screw-topped jars and
seal well. Serve with cold meats or flans.

Total CHO   *180g*
Total calories 750

Spiced Vinegar

550ml/1 pint malt vinegar
3 × 5ml spoons/3 teaspoons pickling
  spice

Warm the vinegar gently in a saucepan, then steep the spice
in it overnight. Use as required.

Total CHO   *neg*
Total calories neg

Cucumber and Onion Raita

1/2 small cucumber, chopped
1 medium onion, chopped
150g/5.3 oz natural yoghurt (1 small
  carton
1 × 5ml spoon/1 teaspoon curry powder

salt, pepper

Garnish
paprika

Mix all the ingredients together well. Sprinkle with paprika and
chill in a refrigerator. Serve with curries and other spicy
dishes.

Total CHO   *20g*
Total calories 140

Spicy Sauerkraut

350g/12 oz sauerkraut, frozen **or**
  canned
2 large carrots, grated
2 stalks celery, trimmed and chopped
1 large onion, chopped

2 medium green peppers, deseeded and
  chopped
1 × 2.5ml spoon/½ teaspoon dill
  seeds
salt, pepper
150ml/¼ pint wine vinegar

Mix the vegetables, dill and seasoning with the wine vinegar.
Marinate for at least 6 hours before serving. Serve hot or cold,
with savoury flans or burgers.

Total CHO   40g
Total calories 200

Dressings

Apple Vinaigrette

150ml/¼ pint white wine vinegar
juice of 1 lemon
1 × 5ml spoon/1 teaspoon made
  French mustard
150ml/¼ pint unsweetened apple juice

1 × 2.5ml spoon/½ teaspoon celery salt
1 clove of garlic, crushed
1 small carrot, grated
salt, pepper

Put the vinegar, lemon juice, mustard, apple juice and celery
salt through a sieve, or process in a blender. Pour into a
screw-topped jar and add the garlic, carrot and seasoning.

Total CHO   20g
Total calories   80

Caraway Dressing

150ml/¼ pint wine vinegar
1 clove of garlic, crushed
1 × 2.5ml spoon/½ teaspoon caraway
  seeds
1 × 5ml spoon/1 teaspoon chives,
  chopped

1 × 5ml spoon/1 teaspoon made
  French mustard
salt, pepper

Mix all the ingredients together well, and leave to stand
for at least 6 hours before serving.

Total CHO   neg
Total calories neg

Carrot Cream Dressing

2 large carrots, sliced
150g/5.3 oz natural yoghurt (1 small
  carton)
1 × 5ml spoon/1 teaspoon curry powder

juice of 1 lemon
salt, freshly ground black pepper
liquid sweetener

Steam the carrots until tender, and pass through a sieve or process in a blender. Mix the purée well with the remaining ingredients. Chill in a refrigerator, and serve as a party dip, or serve with cottage cheese and green salad.

Total CHO   ***30g***
Total calories   ***180***

Cauliflower Dressing

½ small cauliflower, trimmed
1 × 15ml spoon/1 tablespoon wine
  vinegar
150g/5.3 oz natural yoghurt (1 small
  carton)

1 × 5ml spoon/1 teaspoon made
  English mustard

Steam the cauliflower until tender, and pass through a sieve or process in a blender. Mix the purée well with the remaining ingredients, and heat gently. Serve hot over vegetables.

Total CHO   ***10g***
Total calories   ***90***

Chopped Egg Dressing

3 × 15ml spoons/3 tablespoons wine
  vinegar
1 clove of garlic, crushed
1 × 5ml spoon/1 teaspoon made
  English mustard

salt, pepper
1 size 3 egg, hard-boiled and separated

Mix together the vinegar, garlic, mustard, salt and pepper, and add this to the egg yolk. Chop the egg white very finely and mix all the ingredients together well. Serve with salads.

Total CHO   ***neg***
Total calories   ***80***

Dijon Dressing

150ml/¼ pint cider vinegar
Dijon mustard
juice of 1 lemon

2 × 5ml spoons/2 teaspoons skimmed
  milk
salt, pepper

Put all the ingredients in a jug and mix well together with a
fork. Cover, and chill in a refrigerator for 24 hours. Stir well
before serving. Serve with any salads.

Total CHO   **neg**
Total calories **neg**

Horseradish and Yoghurt Dressing

150g/5.3 oz natural yoghurt (1 small
  carton)
2 × 15ml spoons/2 tablespoons
  horseradish, finely grated

salt, pepper

Mix together the yoghurt and horseradish, and season to
taste. Serve with cold meats.

Total CHO   **10g**
Total calories **80**

Mango Dressing

225g/8 oz cottage cheese
juice of 1 lime
1 mango, peeled, stoned and sliced

Mix together all the ingredients and process in a blender.
Serve with salads and seafood.

Total CHO   **30g**
Total calories **350**

Spicy Dressing

2 × 15ml spoons/2 tablespoons
  skimmed milk
1 egg white
1 × 5ml spoon/1 teaspoon made
  English mustard

150ml/¼ pint cold water
150ml/¼ pint wine vinegar
1 clove of garlic, crushed
salt, pepper

Mix all the ingredients together well and serve with salads.

Total CHO   **neg**
Total calories   **20**

Tofu Dressing

200g/7 oz soya bean curd (tofu)
juice of 1 lemon
1 size 3 egg, hard-boiled and chopped
1 × 5ml spoon/1 teaspoon made
  French mustard

150g/5.3 oz natural yoghurt (1 small
  carton)
2 × 15ml spoons/2 tablespoons wine
  vinegar
salt, pepper

Mix all the ingredients together well. Pass through a sieve or
process in a blender to form a smooth cream. Serve cold with
mixed salads or hot vegetables.

Total CHO   **20g**
Total calories   **360**

Vinaigrette

150ml/¼ pint wine vinegar
juice of 1 lemon
salt, pepper

Mix all the ingredients together well, and use for any green
salad.

Total CHO   **neg**
Total calories   **neg**

Yoghurt Dressing (1)

150g/5.3 oz natural yoghurt (1 small
  carton)
1 × 5ml spoon/1 teaspoon made
  French mustard

2 × 15ml spoons/2 tablespoons wine
  vinegar
juice of 1 lemon
salt, pepper

Mix all the ingredients together well, and serve with fish,
eggs or cold chicken.

Total CHO	**10g**
Total calories	**80**

Yoghurt Dressing (2)

150g/5.3 oz natural yoghurt (1 small
  carton)
2 × 15ml spoons/2 tablespoons wine
  vinegar

salt, pepper

Mix all the ingredients together well and serve with fish, eggs
or cold chicken.

Total CHO	**10g**
Total calories	**80**

Mock Mayonnaise

100g/4 oz cottage cheese
1 × 15ml spoon/1 tablespoon wine
  vinegar
1 × 5ml spoon/1 teaspoon made
  French mustard
juice of ½ lemon

150g/5.3 oz natural yoghurt (1 small
  carton)
1 × 2.5ml spoon/½ teaspoon garlic salt
1 × 2.5ml spoon/½ teaspoon celery salt
freshly ground black pepper

Mix all the ingredients together well, and sieve, or process in
a blender. Pour into a screw-topped jar.
Note This mayonnaise needs to be stirred well before using
a second time.

Total CHO	**10g**
Total calories	**180**

Wholewheat Pasta Salad (Page 79)

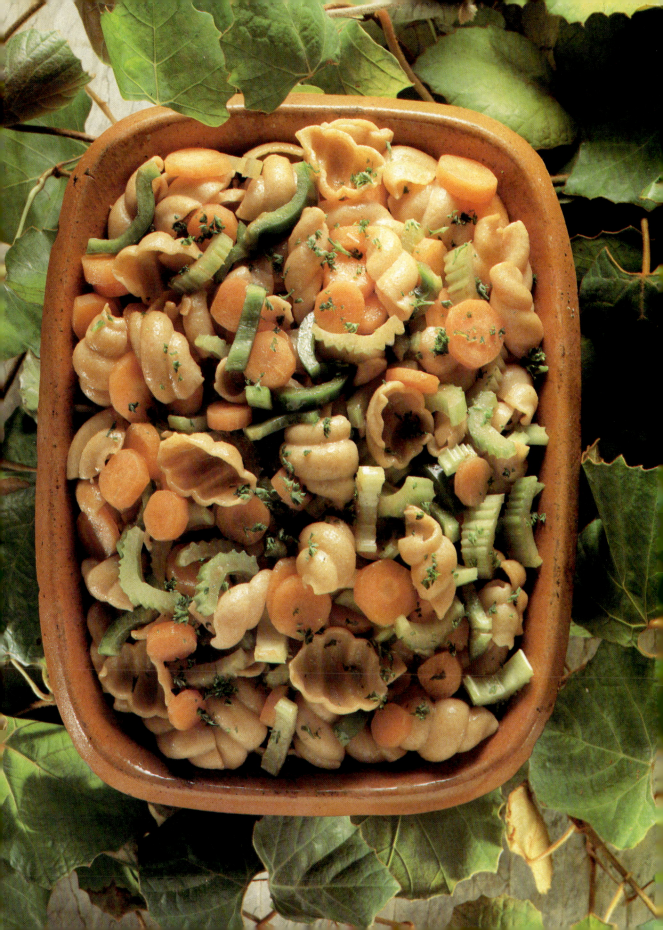

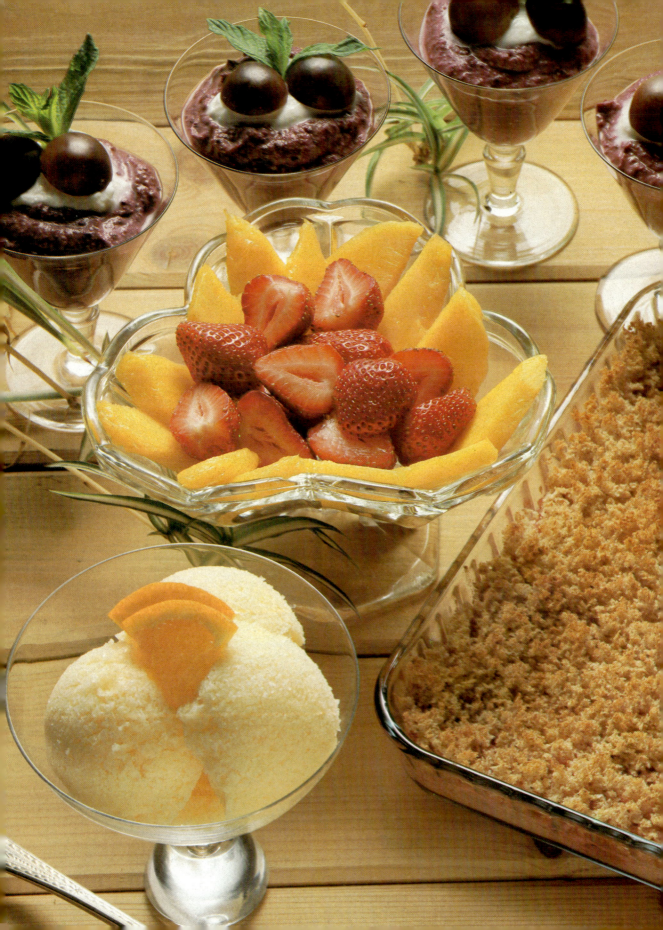

Sauces

Cucumber Sauce

$1/2$ small cucumber, peeled and chopped
150ml/$1/4$ pint wine vinegar
salt, pepper

Mix together the ingredients, then sieve, or process in a blender. Serve with white fish.

Total CHO   **neg**
Total calories   **25**

Green Pepper Sauce

275ml/$1/2$ pint skimmed milk
1 × 15ml spoon/1 tablespoon arrowroot
1 × 15ml spoon/1 tablespoon low fat spread

$1/2$ small green pepper, deseeded and chopped
1 × 5ml spoon/1 teaspoon soy sauce
salt, pepper

Put the milk, arrowroot and spread in a saucepan. Heat gently to boiling point, stirring all the time. Reduce the heat, add the pepper, soy sauce and seasoning, and simmer for a further 5 minutes. Serve hot with meat or fish.

Variation
Use a red pepper instead of a green pepper.

Total CHO   **25g**
Total calories   **150**

A Selection of Desserts
Blackcurrant Dessert (page 123), Mangoes and Strawberries (page 125), Yoghurt Orange Ice (page 129) and *Raspberry Curd Crumble (page 109)*

Horseradish and Apple Sauce

1 medium cooking apple, peeled and
 cored
2 × 15ml spoons / 2 tablespoons
 horseradish, grated

Steam the apple until tender, then mash together with the grated horseradish. Serve hot or cold with roast beef.

Total CHO   15g
Total calories   60

Sauce Provençale

150g / 5.3 oz natural yoghurt (1 small
 carton)
2 × 15ml spoons / 2 tablespoons wine
 vinegar
4 × 15ml spoons / 4 tablespoons
 concentrated tomato purée

1 clove of garlic, crushed
1 × 2.5ml spoon / ½ teaspoon thyme
salt, pepper

Mix all the ingredients together well, and serve cold with fish or cold chicken.

Total CHO   15g
Total calories   110

Slim Salad Sauce

275ml / ½ pint tomato juice
2 × 15ml spoons / 2 tablespoons wine
 vinegar
½ small green pepper, deseeded and
 chopped
salt, pepper

1 × 2.5ml spoon / ½ teaspoon garlic
 powder
1 × 5ml spoon / 1 teaspoon made
 English mustard
1 × 15ml spoon / 1 tablespoon
 Worcestershire sauce

Put all the ingredients in a saucepan. Heat to boiling point, reduce the heat, cover and simmer for 30 minutes. Season to taste, and pour into a serving jug. Serve hot or cold with meat and poultry.

Total CHO   15g
Total calories   60

Spinach Sauce

225g/8 oz frozen spinach
150ml/¼ pint skimmed milk
75g/3 oz natural yoghurt

1 × 2.5ml spoon/½ teaspoon grated
  nutmeg
salt, pepper

Cook the spinach in boiling salted water for 5 minutes. Drain well, and sieve, or process in a blender. Mix in the milk, yoghurt and nutmeg, and season to taste. Serve with white fish.

Total CHO   20g
Total calories 140

Tartare Sauce

150g/5.3 oz natural yoghurt (1 small
  carton)
1 × 15ml spoon/1 tablespoon wine
  vinegar

1 × 5ml spoon/1 teaspoon chives,
  chopped
1 × 5ml spoon/1 teaspoon capers,
  chopped
salt, pepper

Mix all the ingredients together well, and serve with fish.

Total CHO   10g
Total calories   80

Tomato Sauce (1)

1 × 400g/14 oz can tomatoes
2 medium onions, finely chopped
2 cloves garlic, crushed
2 × 15ml spoons/2 tablespoons vinegar

1 × 2.5ml spoon/½ teaspoon oregano
1 × 2.5ml spoon/½ teaspoon basil
1 × 2.5ml spoon/½ teaspoon coriander
salt, pepper

Put all the ingredients in a large saucepan. Heat to boiling point, reduce the heat, cover and simmer for 45 minutes. Sieve, or process in a blender. Leave to stand for 24 hours before serving. Season to taste, and use cold as a salad dressing, or re-heat and serve hot.

Total CHO   20g
Total calories 100

Tomato Sauce (2)

450g/1 lb tomatoes, chopped
1 large onion, finely chopped
2 cloves garlic, crushed
2 × 15ml spoons/2 tablespoons vinegar

1 × 5ml spoon/1 teaspoon oregano
1 × 5ml spoon/1 teaspoon basil
salt, freshly ground black pepper

Put all the ingredients in a saucepan. Heat to boiling point, reduce the heat, cover and simmer for 30 minutes. Sieve, or process in a blender and leave to stand for 24 hours. Use cold as a salad dressing, or re-heat and serve hot.

Total CHO   20g
Total calories 100

Yoghurt Sauce

1 × 15ml spoon/1 tablespoon natural
  yoghurt
1 × 5ml spoon/1 teaspoon made
  French mustard

juice of 1 lemon
1 × 2.5ml spoon/½ teaspoon garlic salt
salt, pepper

Mix all the ingredients together well. This sauce is ideal as a topping for fish steaks, salads or hard-boiled eggs.

Total CHO   neg
Total calories 10

Puddings, Desserts and Home Baking

As few people can resist the occasional old-fashioned pudding, rich dessert or home-baked cake, a number of recipes based on these have been included. These combine ingredients which are relatively low in calories to produce unusual flavours and textures. Although their fat content has been kept to a minimum, none are low enough in calories to be eaten in quantity.

Hot Puddings

Apple Meringue

2 medium cooking apples
2 size 3 eggs, separated
2 × 15ml spoons/2 tablespoons sultanas

Remove the apple cores so as to leave a hole in which to pour the egg yolks. Put the apples in an ovenproof dish. Beat the yolks together with the sultanas and pour into the fruit. Whisk the egg whites until stiff and use to top each apple. Cook at 190°C/375°F/Gas 5 for 25 minutes until the meringue is set. Serve immediately.

Serves 2

Total CHO   **40g**
Total calories **320**

Baked Apple

2 medium cooking apples, cored
2 large prunes, stoned
liquid sweetener

2 × 5ml spoons/2 teaspoons natural
 yoghurt

Put the apples on a baking tray and place a prune and two drops of liquid sweetener in each apple. Cook at 190°C/375°F/Gas 5 for 25 minutes. Serve hot with 1 × 5ml spoon/1 teaspoon of yoghurt on top of each apple.

Serves 2

Total CHO   **40g**
Total calories **200**

Baked Grapefruit

1 very large grapefruit
2 × 5ml spoons/2 teaspoons fructose
1 × 2.5ml spoon/½ teaspoon ground
  coriander
1 × 2.5ml spoon/½ teaspoon cinnamon

Decoration
sprigs of fresh mint

Cut the grapefruit in half crossways, and sprinkle with the
fructose, coriander and cinnamon. Place the two halves
together and wrap with foil. Cook at 190°C/375°F/Gas 5 for
15 minutes. Decorate the grapefruit halves with sprigs of fresh
mint.

Serves 2

Total CHO   10g
Total calories 100

Lime Baked Pears

2 large pears, peeled
2 cloves
150ml/¼ pint low-calorie lime juice
liquid sweetener

Decoration
grated lemon rind

Cut the pears in half lengthways and put them in a deep
ovenproof dish with the cloves and lime juice. Cover with foil
and cook at 190°C/375°F/Gas 5 for 40 minutes. Remove the
cloves, add the liquid sweetener and decorate with a little
grated lemon rind.

Serves 2

Total CHO   20g
Total calories 100

Slimmer's Rice Pudding

425ml/¾ pint skimmed milk
25g/1 oz brown rice flakes

liquid sweetener
grated nutmeg

Put the skimmed milk in a saucepan, and heat to boiling point.
Add the rice flakes, reduce the heat, cover and simmer for 5
minutes. Remove from the heat, add the liquid sweetener, and
sprinkle with nutmeg.

Serves 2

Total CHO   40g
Total calories 220

Date and Banana Pudding

75g/3 oz pitted dried dates
juice of 1 lemon
2 × 15ml spoons/2 tablespoons cold
  water
2 small bananas
100g/4 oz rolled oats

1 size 3 egg, well beaten
150ml/¼ pint skimmed milk
liquid sweetener
2 × 5ml spoons/2 teaspoons mixed
  spice

Put the dates in a saucepan with the lemon juice and water, and cook gently for about 5 minutes. Place in an ovenproof dish. Mash one banana, and mix together with the oats, egg, milk, liquid sweetener and the mixed spice. Spread over the dates and bake at 180°C/350°F/Gas 4 for 25 minutes. Slice the remaining banana and use to decorate the pudding. Serve immediately.

Serves 4

Total CHO   140g
Total calories   760

Date Crumble

100g/4 oz pitted dried dates
3 × 15ml spoons/3 tablespoons cold
  water
100g/4 oz rolled oats

juice of 1 large lemon
1 × 5ml spoon/1 teaspoon grated
  nutmeg

Put the dates in a saucepan with the water and cook gently for about 5 minutes. Place in a small ovenproof dish and cover with the rolled oats. Sprinkle the lemon juice and nutmeg over the top and bake at 190°C/375°F/Gas 5 for 25 minutes. Serve hot.

Serves 4

Total CHO   140g
Total calories   660

Raspberry Curd Crumble

350g/12 oz raspberries
liquid sweetener
100g/4 oz curd cheese

50g/2 oz fresh wholemeal breadcrumbs
1 × 2.5ml spoon/½ teaspoon cinnamon
1 × 2.5ml spoon/½ teaspoon nutmeg

Put the raspberries in a bowl, add the liquid sweetener and fold in the curd cheese. Put the mixture into a 550ml/1 pint ovenproof dish, cover with the breadcrumbs and sprinkle with cinnamon and nutmeg. Bake at 220°C/425°F/Gas 7 for 10 minutes. Serve hot or cold.

Serves 4

Total CHO   40g
Total calories   340

Lemon and Apricot Flan

100g/4 oz dried apricots
100g/4 oz wholemeal/wholewheat flour
50g/2 oz low fat spread
1 × 5ml spoon/1 teaspoon arrowroot
150g/5.3 oz natural yoghurt (1 small
  carton)

grated rind and juice of 1 lemon
liquid sweetener

Decoration
3 fresh apricots, stoned and halved

Soak the dried apricots in water overnight, then cook gently for 10 minutes in a little boiling water.

Rub together the flour and spread until the mixture resembles fine breadcrumbs. Add a little water and mix to form a soft dough. Roll out, and use the pastry to line a 20cm/8 inch flan ring. Leave in a refrigerator for at least 15 minutes. Bake the pastry case blind at 180°C/350°F/Gas 4 for 20 minutes.

Mix the arrowroot with a little cold water and combine with the apricots, yoghurt, lemon rind and juice, and liquid sweetener. Pour into the pastry case and bake at 180°C/350°F/Gas 4 for a further 25 minutes. Decorate with the apricot halves.

Total CHO   140g
Total calories   740

Oaty Plum Pie

450g/1 lb dessert plums, stoned
liquid sweetener
100g/4 oz rolled oats
25g/1 oz sultanas
25g/1 oz wholewheat flakes (breakfast
  cereal)

1 × 5ml spoon/1 teaspoon nutmeg
1 size 3 egg, well beaten
150ml/¼ pint skimmed milk

Decoration
1 × 5ml spoon/1 teaspoon cinnamon

Put the plums and liquid sweetener in a large saucepan with a little cold water. Heat to boiling point, reduce the heat, cover and simmer for 10 minutes. Pour into an ovenproof dish. Mix the remaining ingredients together well and pour over the plums. Bake at 190°C/375°F/Gas 5 for 25 minutes. Sprinkle with cinnamon and serve hot.

Serves 4

Total CHO   160g
Total calories   840

Serving suggestion Natural yoghurt

Rhubarb Bake

450g/1 lb rhubarb, trimmed and
  chopped
liquid sweetener
175g/6 oz fresh wholemeal
  breadcrumbs

1 × 15ml spoon/1 tablespoon fructose
25g/1 oz sultanas
2 size 3 eggs, well beaten

Steam the rhubarb for about 15 minutes until tender. Mix with the liquid sweetener and pour into an ovenproof dish. Mix together the breadcrumbs, fructose and sultanas, and bind together with the beaten egg. Spread over the top of the rhubarb and bake at 180°C/350°F/Gas 4 for 25 minutes. Serve hot or cold.

Serves 4

Total CHO   120g
Total calories   760

Sultana Banana Bake

150g/5.3 oz natural yoghurt (1 small
  carton)
4 small bananas, mashed
25g/1 oz low fat spread
100g/4 oz wholemeal/wholewheat
  self- raising flour

25g/1 oz fructose
25g/1 oz sultanas
1 × 5ml spoon/1 teaspoon cinnamon
1 × 5ml spoon/1 teaspoon nutmeg

Mix together the yoghurt and bananas and put in an ovenproof dish. Rub the spread into the flour until the mixture resembles fine breadcrumbs. Stir in the fructose, sultanas, cinnamon and nutmeg. Cover the banana and yoghurt mixture with this topping and bake at 190°C/375°F/Gas 5 for 25 minutes. Serve hot or cold.

Serves 4

Total CHO   140g
Total calories   820

Egg Custard

425ml/¾ pint skimmed milk
2 size 3 eggs, well beaten
grated nutmeg

Mix together the milk and eggs. Pour into a baking dish, sprinkle with the nutmeg and bake at 190°C/375°F/Gas 5 for about 1 hour or until set.

Serves 4
Total CHO   20g
Total calories   280

Pouring Custard

4 × 15ml spoons/4 tablespoons custard
 powder
550ml/1 pint skimmed milk
liquid sweetener

Mix the custard powder with a little of the milk. Heat the
remaining milk, and before it reaches boiling point, stir in the
custard paste. Simmer until the custard thickens, stirring all
the time. Cook for a further 3 minutes, remove from the heat
and stir in the liquid sweetener. Use as required.

Total CHO   *70g*
Total calories *330*

Hot Yoghurt Cake

50g/2 oz low fat spread
liquid sweetener
175g/6 oz fresh wholemeal
 breadcrumbs, toasted
1 × 5ml spoon/1 teaspoon arrowroot
2 × 15ml spoons/2 tablespoons cold
 water

150g/5.3 oz natural yoghurt (1 small
 carton)
2 size 3 eggs, well beaten
1 × 5ml spoon/1 teaspoon vanilla
 essence
25g/1 oz raisins

Melt the spread in a saucepan, then stir in the liquid
sweetener and the breadcrumbs. Press the mixture on to the
base of a 20cm/8 inch loose-bottomed cake tin lined with
greaseproof paper, and chill in a refrigerator.

Meanwhile, mix the arrowroot with the cold water and
yoghurt. Put in a double saucepan and heat very gently to
boiling point. Remove from the heat and leave to cool. Add
the eggs, vanilla essence and raisins, and mix together well.
Pour the yoghurt mixture over the chilled breadcrumb base.
Bake at 180°C/350°F/Gas 4 for 20 minutes or until the
mixture has set, then remove from the tin carefully.
Note This cake will keep for a week if stored covered in a
 refrigerator.

Total CHO   *90g*
Total calories *750*

Spicy-topped Pears

2 large pears, peeled
juice of 1 lemon
1 size 3 egg, well beaten
6 × 15ml spoons/6 tablespoons
  skimmed milk
100g/4 oz curd cheese

liquid sweetener
1 × 5ml spoon/1 teaspoon ground
  ginger
4 × 15ml spoons/4 tablespoons
  wholewheat flakes (breakfast cereal)

Cut the pears in half lengthways and rub all over with the lemon juice. Beat together the egg, milk, curd cheese and liquid sweetener. Place the pears on a baking tray and fill each half with the mixture. Sprinkle with the ginger and cereal and bake at 190°C/375°F/Gas 5 for 20 minutes. Serve hot or cold.

Serves 4

Total CHO   40g
Total calories   360

Desserts

Green Mountain Cream

2 × 15ml spoons/2 tablespoons water
3 × 5ml spoons/3 teaspoons gelatine
425ml/¾ pint water
3 × 15ml spoons/3 tablespoons
  sugar-free/low calorie lime cordial
1 × 15ml spoon/1 tablespoon lemon
  juice
green food colouring

liquid sweetener
150g/5.3 oz natural yoghurt (1 small
  carton)
75g/3 oz cottage cheese
75g/3 oz quark cheese

Decoration
fresh mint leaves

Put the 2 × 15ml spoons/2 tablespoons water in a heatproof container, sprinkle on the gelatine and leave to soften. Stand the container in a pan of hot water and stir until the gelatine dissolves. Mix with the remaining water, the lime cordial, lemon juice, food colouring and liquid sweetener. Leave in a refrigerator until set.

Mix together the yoghurt and cheeses, and add liquid sweetener to taste. Fold into the jelly to create a marbled effect. Chill in a refrigerator, and serve decorated with mint leaves.

Serves 2

Total CHO   10g
Total calories   220

Blackcurrant Jelly

2 × 15ml spoons/2 tablespoons water
3 × 5ml spoons/3 teaspoons gelatine
425ml/¾ pint water
3 × 15ml spoons/3 tablespoons
 sugar-free/low calorie blackcurrant
 cordial

1 × 15ml spoon/1 tablespoon lemon
 juice
liquid sweetener

Decoration
fresh blackcurrants

Put the 2 × 15ml spoons/2 tablespoons water in a heatproof container, sprinkle in the gelatine and leave to soften. Stand the container in a pan of hot water and stir until the gelatine dissolves. Mix with the remaining ingredients. Pour into a glass serving dish and leave in a refrigerator until set. Decorate with fresh blackcurrants.

Serves 2

Total CHO   *neg*
Total calories   *20*

Variation
Substitute lime cordial for the blackcurrant cordial, and add a few drops of green food colouring. Decorate with lemon slices.

Total CHO   *neg*
Total calories   *10*

Summer Strawberries

2 × 15ml spoons/2 tablespoons water
3 × 5ml spoons/3 teaspoons gelatine
350g/12 oz strawberries, hulled
150ml/¼ pint skimmed milk

liquid sweetener

Decoration
fresh strawberries, halved

Put the water into a heatproof container, sprinkle in the gelatine and leave to soften. Stand the container in a pan of hot water and stir until the gelatine dissolves. Mix together with the strawberries, milk and liquid sweetener, and sieve, or process in a blender. Pour into a glass serving bowl and leave to set in a refrigerator. When set, decorate with a few halved strawberries.

Serves 2

Total CHO   *30g*
Total calories   *140*

Variation
Use 450g/1 lb raspberries instead of the strawberries and increase the skimmed milk to 275ml/½ pint.

Total CHO   *40g*
Total calories   *200*

Banana Crunch

150g/5.3 oz natural yoghurt (1 small carton)
25g/1 oz wholewheat flakes (breakfast cereal)
1 small banana, sliced

25g/1 oz almonds, chopped

Decoration
wholewheat flakes (breakfast cereal)

Mix all the ingredients together well, and put the mixture into two glass dishes. Chill in a refrigerator before serving. Decorate with a sprinkling of wholewheat flakes.

Serves 2
Total CHO   40g
Total calories   360

Yoghurt Egg Fluff

2 size 3 eggs, separated
2 × 5ml spoons/2 teaspoons fructose
2 × 15ml spoons/2 tablespoons water

3 × 5ml spoons/3 teaspoons gelatine
juice and grated rind of 1 lemon
5 × 15ml spoons/5 tablespoons natural yoghurt

Put the egg yolks and fructose in a bowl over a pan of boiling water and whisk until the mixture thickens. Remove from the heat and continue whisking until cool. Put the water into a heatproof container, sprinkle in the gelatine and leave to soften. Stand the container in a pan of hot water and stir until the gelatine dissolves. Fold the lemon rind and juice, the yoghurt and gelatine into the egg mixture. Whisk the egg whites until very stiff and fold into the mixture. Pour into two tall glasses and leave to set in a refrigerator.

Serves 2

Total CHO   neg
Total calories   240

Prune Delight

100g/4 oz stoned prunes
2 × 15ml spoons/2 tablespoons water
3 × 5ml spoons/3 teaspoons gelatine

vanilla essence
2 size 3 egg whites

Serves 2

Soak the prunes overnight in cold water. Drain, and put in a saucepan with sufficient boiling water to cover, and cook gently for 5 minutes. Sieve, or process in a blender. Put the water into a heatproof container, sprinkle in the gelatine and leave to soften. Stand the container in a pan of hot water and stir until the gelatine dissolves. Mix together with the prune purée and a few drops of vanilla essence. Whisk the egg whites until very stiff and gently fold into the prune mixture. Pour into two tall sundae glasses and leave to set in a refrigerator.

Total CHO   40g
Total calories   180

Snow Cream

2 × 15ml spoons/2 tablespoons water
3 × 5ml spoons/3 teaspoons gelatine
150ml/¼ pint sugar-free/low calorie
  orange drink
150ml/¼ pint water
1 × 15ml spoon/1 tablespoon lemon
  juice
orange food colouring

liquid sweetener
4 × 15ml spoons/4 tablespoons
  skimmed milk
100g/4 oz cottage cheese

Decoration
fresh mint leaves

Serves 2

Put the 2 × 15ml spoons/2 tablespoons water in a heatproof container, sprinkle in the gelatine and leave to soften. Stand the container in a pan of hot water and stir until the gelatine dissolves. Mix together with the orange drink, the remaining water, lemon juice, food colour and liquid sweetener, and leave to set in a refrigerator. When set solid, chop the jelly into cubes. Place on a flat serving dish, making a well in the centre. Mix together the milk, cottage cheese and sweetener and pour into the well. Decorate with fresh mint.

Total CHO   neg
Total calories   120

Apricot Fluff

350g/12 oz fresh apricots **or** 50g/2 oz
dried apricots, chopped
2 × 15ml spoons/2 tablespoons water

3 × 5ml spoons/3 teaspoons gelatine
2 egg whites

Cook the apricots in a little water until tender, then process in
a blender. Put the water in a heatproof container, sprinkle in
the gelatine and leave to soften. Stand the container in a pan
of hot water and stir until the gelatine dissolves. Stir into the
apricot purée. Whisk the egg whites until stiff and gently fold
into the apricot mixture. Pour into two sundae glasses and
leave in a refrigerator to set.

Serves 2

Total CHO   20g
Total calories 120

Apricot Compôte

1 × 225g/8 oz can apricots in natural
juice
4 cloves
1 cinnamon stick

150g/5.3 oz natural yoghurt (1 small
carton)
liquid sweetener
2 × 15ml spoons/2 tablespoons
wholewheat flakes (breakfast cereal)

Put the apricots, their juice and the cloves and cinnamon in a
saucepan and cook gently for 10 minutes. Remove the cloves
and cinnamon stick, leave to cool, then stir in the yoghurt and
liquid sweetener. Chill in a refrigerator and sprinkle with
cereal before serving.

Serves 2

Total CHO   40g
Total calories 200

Apple Jelly

2 × 15ml spoons/2 tablespoons water
4 × 5ml spoons/4 teaspoons gelatine
550ml/1 pint apple juice
1 × 15ml spoon/1 tablespoon lemon
juice

liquid sweetener
green food colouring

Decoration
lemon twists

Put the water into a heatproof container, sprinkle in the
gelatine and leave to soften. Stand the container in a pan of
hot water and stir until the gelatine dissolves. Mix with the
apple juice, lemon juice, liquid sweetener and a few drops of
food colouring, then pour into a glass serving dish and leave
to set in a refrigerator. When set, decorate with lemon twists.

Serves 4

Total CHO   60g
Total calories 220

Bramley Cinnamon Snow

900g/2 lb Bramley apples, peeled, cored
  and sliced
3 pitted dried dates, finely chopped
grated rind and juice of 1 lemon

liquid sweetener
2 egg whites
2 × 5ml spoons/2 teaspoons cinnamon

Steam the apples gently for about 15 minutes until tender.
Add the dates, lemon rind and juice and liquid sweetener.
Increase the heat, cover and cook for a further 5 minutes,
stirring frequently. Leave to cool completely. Whisk the egg
whites until stiff and fold into the cold apple purée. Serve in
individual glass dishes and sprinkle with cinnamon.

Serves 4

Total CHO   80g
Total calories 320

Apricot Soufflé

175g/6 oz dried apricots
2 size 3 eggs, separated
25g/1 oz fructose
150ml/¼ pint cold water
3 × 5ml spoons/3 teaspoons gelatine

150g/5.3 oz natural yoghurt (1 small
  carton)
juice of 1 lemon

Decoration
dried apricots, chopped

Prepare a 15cm/6 inch souffle dish, making a 5cm/2 inch
collar. Put the apricots in a saucepan with sufficient boiling
water to cover. Cook until tender, then sieve, or process in a
blender.

   Put the egg yolks and fructose in a bowl over boiling water,
and beat for about 5 minutes until the mixture thickens and
becomes paler. Remove from the heat and continue beating
until the mixture is cool.

   Put the water into a heatproof container, sprinkle in the
gelatine and leave to soften. Stand the container in a pan of
hot water and stir until the gelatine dissolves. Leave to cool
slightly, and fold into the egg mixture. Fold in the yoghurt,
apricot purée and lemon juice. Whisk the egg whites until very
stiff and fold into the mixture. Pour into the soufflé dish and
leave to set in a refrigerator.

   Carefully remove the collar and decorate the soufflé with a
few chopped, dried apricots.

Serves 4

Total CHO   80g
Total calories 660

Raisin Wheat Bread (page 135)

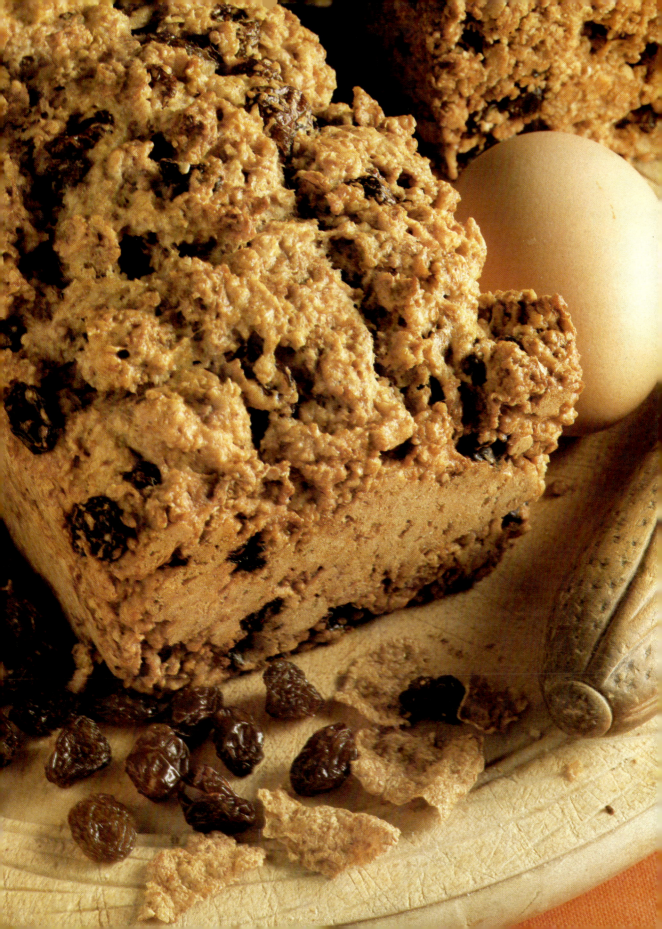

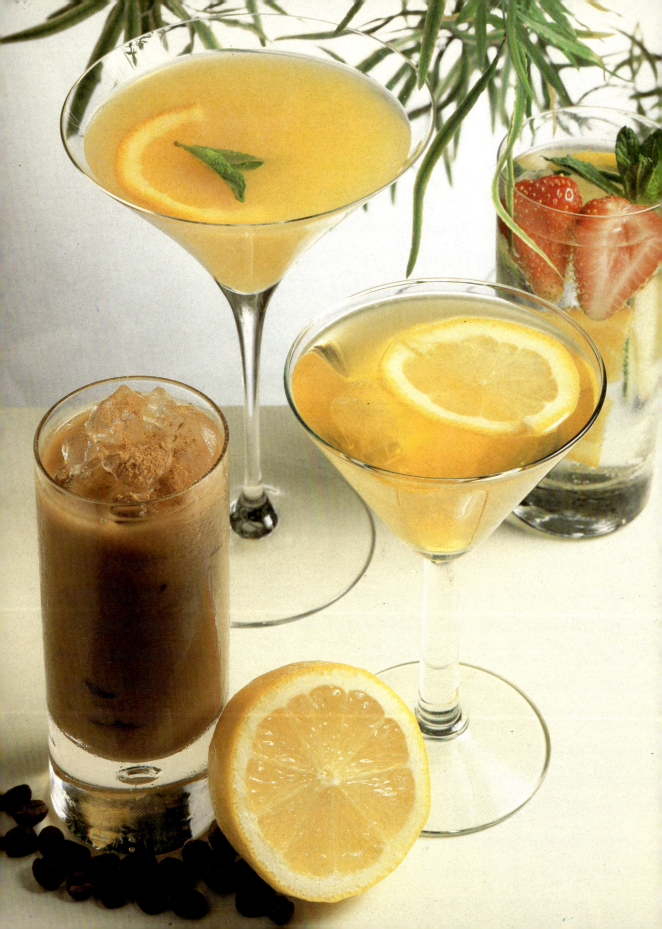

Banana and Ricotta Fool

2 × 15ml spoons/2 tablespoons water
3 × 5ml spoons/3 teaspoons gelatine
6 × 15ml spoons/6 tablespoons natural
 orange juice
1 large banana

150g/5.3 oz natural yoghurt (1 small
 carton)
100g/4 oz Ricotta cheese
juice of ½ lemon
1 × 2.5ml spoon/½ teaspoon nutmeg
liquid sweetener

Put the water into a heatproof container, sprinkle in the gelatine and leave to soften. Stand the container in a pan of hot water and stir until the gelatine dissolves. Chop most of the banana and reserve a few slices for decoration. Mix the chopped banana with the other ingredients, then sieve, or process in a blender. Pour into four glass dishes and leave to set in a refrigerator.Decorate with the reserved banana slices.

Serves 4

Total CHO **40g**
Total calories **640**

Blackberry and Apple Chiffon

350g/12 oz blackberries
450g/1 lb cooking apples, peeled, cored
 and sliced
275ml/½ pint water
liquid sweetener

3 × 5ml spoons/3 teaspoons gelatine
3 × 15ml spoons/3 tablespoons
 skimmed milk

Decoration
blackberries

Put the blackberries and apple in a saucepan with half the water, and cook gently for about 15 minutes. Remove from the heat and add the liquid sweetener. Put the remaining water in a heatproof container, sprinkle in the gelatine and leave to soften. Stand the container in a pan of hot water and stir until the gelatine dissolves. Stir into the fruit mixture with the skimmed milk. Pour into a serving dish and leave to set in a refrigerator. When set, decorate the top with a few blackberries.

Serves 4

Total CHO **60g**
Total calories **260**

A Selection of Drinks
At the back, Orange and Grapefruit Cocktail (page 139) and Slimmer's Fruit Punch (page 140)
At the front, Chilled Coffee Cup (page 137) and Crazy Cocktail (page 138)

Blackberry and Apple Mousse

2 × 15ml spoons/2 tablespoons water
3 × 5ml spoons/3 teaspoons gelatine
450g/1 lb cooking apples, peeled, cored
    and cooked
225g/8 oz blackberries
150ml/¼ pint skimmed milk

liquid sweetener

Decoration
2 × 15ml spoons/2 tablespoons
    wholewheat flakes (breakfast cereal)

Put the water in a heatproof container, sprinkle in the gelatine and leave to soften. Stand the heatproof container in a pan of hot water and stir until the gelatine dissolves. Mix with the apple, blackberries, milk and liquid sweetener. Sieve, or process in a blender. Pour into a 550ml/1 pint mould and leave to set in a refrigerator. Sprinkle with the cereal before serving.

Serves 4

Total CHO   60g
Total calories 280

Blackcurrant Mousse

450g/1 lb blackcurrants
2 × 15ml spoons/2 tablespoons cold
    water
3 × 5ml spoons/3 teaspoons gelatine
150g/5.3 oz natural yoghurt (1 small
    carton)

50g/2 oz cottage cheese
2 egg whites
liquid sweetener

Cook the blackcurrants in a little water, and leave to cool. Put the water in a heatproof container, sprinkle in the gelatine and leave to soften. Stand the container in a pan of hot water and stir until the gelatine dissolves. Mix together with the blackcurrants, yoghurt and cottage cheese. Sieve, or process in a blender. Whisk the egg whites until stiff and fold into the blackcurrant mixture with the liquid sweetener. Pour into a serving bowl and leave in a refrigerator to set.

Serves 4

Total CHO   40g
Total calories 280

Blackcurrant Dessert

225g/8 oz blackcurrants
100g/4 oz cottage cheese
liquid sweetener
juice of 1/2 lemon

Decoration
4 × 5ml spoons/4 tablespoons natural
  yoghurt
black grapes, halved
mint leaves

Steam the blackcurrants for about 10 minutes until tender. Stir in the cheese, sweetener and lemon juice. Sieve, or process in a blender. Pour into four glass dishes and chill in a refrigerator before serving. Put a spoonful of yoghurt in each glass dish, and decorate with a grape half and mint leaves.

Serves 4

Total CHO   ***20g***
Total calories ***180***

English Plums

450g/1 lb dessert plums, stoned
1 cinnamon stick
juice of 1 lemon
3 × 15ml spoons/3 tablespoons cold
  water

1 × 2.5ml spoon/1/2 teaspoon mixed
  spice
liquid sweetener

Accompaniment
natural yoghurt

Put all the ingredients in a large saucepan. Heat to boiling point, reduce the heat, cover and simmer for 25 minutes. Leave to cool completely, then remove the cinnamon stick and sieve, or process in a blender. Serve with a spoonful of natural yoghurt.

Serves 4

Total CHO   ***40g***
Total calories ***160***

Cool Spicy Fruit

150g/5.3 oz natural yoghurt (1 small
  carton)
1 × 5ml spoon/1 teaspoon curry powder
liquid sweetener
1/2 medium honeydew melon, skinned
  deseeded and sliced

2 large peaches, sliced
1 small cucumber, peeled and cubed

Decoration
orange segments
cucumber slices

Mix together the yoghurt, curry powder and sweetener. Gently fold in the fruit and cucumber. Chill in a refrigerator before serving. Decorate with orange segments and cucumber slices.

Serves 4
Total CHO   ***40g***
Total calories ***220***

Fruit Compôte

1 large pear, peeled, cored and sliced
1 medium apple, peeled, cored and
 sliced
1 mango, peeled and sliced

1 medium grapefruit, divided into
 segments
10 large black grapes
ground cinnamon

Mix all the fruit together in a large glass bowl. Chill in a
refrigerator for at least 2 hours before serving. Sprinkle
with a little cinnamon.

Serves 4
Total CHO   60g
Total calories 280

Fruit Yoghurt Dessert

1 small grapefruit, peeled and cut into
 chunks
1 large orange, peeled and cut into
 chunks
1 medium apple, cored and sliced
1 medium pear, cored and sliced

150g/5.3 oz natural yoghurt (1 small
 carton)
liquid sweetener

Decoration
sliced strawberries

Mix the fruit together and gently fold in the yoghurt and liquid
sweetener. Chill in a refrigerator, put the mixture into four
glass dishes and decorate with sliced strawberries.

Serves 4
Total CHO   40g
Total calories 220

Gingered Melon Fruit Salad

1 large orange, divided into segments
1 medium red-skinned apple, cored and
 sliced
1 small banana, sliced

450g/1 lb watermelon, skinned
 deseeded and cubed
1 × 5ml spoon/1 teaspoon ground
 ginger

Mix all the fruit together and sprinkle with ginger. Chill in a
refrigerator before serving.

Serves 4
Total CHO   40g
Total calories 180

Tangy Fruit Salad

1 small grapefruit, divided into segments
1 large orange, divided into segments
1 mango, peeled, stoned and sliced

5 × 15ml spoons/5 tablespoons
  sugar-free/low calorie bitter lemon

Mix the fruit gently with the bitter lemon, and chill in a refrigerator for at least 2 hours before serving.

Serves 4
Total CHO **40g**
Total calories **160**

Mangoes and Strawberries

1 large mango peeled, stoned and sliced
225g/8 oz strawberries, hulled and
  halved

Mix together the fruit and chill in a refrigerator. Serve in a glass dish.

Serves 4
Total CHO **40g**
Total calories **160**

Melon Surprise

1 small honeydew melon
1 × 225g/8 oz can pineapple in natural
  juice
2 medium red-skinned apples, cored
  and sliced
1 large orange, divided into segments

juice of 1 orange
liquid sweetener
1 × 5ml spoon/1 teaspoon cinnamon

Decoration
white grapes

Cut the melon in half crossways and scoop out the seeds. Carefully remove the flesh and cut into small cubes. In a large bowl mix together the melon, pineapple, apples, orange, orange juice and liquid sweetener. Put the fruit back into the melon halves, sprinkle with cinnamon and decorate with a few white grapes. Serve one melon half between two people.

Serves 4

Total CHO **80g**
Total calories **320**

Orange Apple Jelly

4 × 15ml spoons/4 tablespoons water
6 × 5ml spoons/6 teaspoons gelatine
150ml/¼ pint unsweetened apple juice
275ml/½ pint unsweetened orange juice
150g/5.3 oz natural yoghurt (1 small
  carton)

liquid sweetener

Decoration
thin orange slices

Put the water in a heatproof container, sprinkle on the gelatine and leave to soften. Stand the container in a pan of hot water and stir until the gelatine dissolves. Mix together with the apple juice, orange juice, yoghurt and liquid sweetener. Pour into individual glass dishes and leave to set in a refrigerator. When set, decorate with orange slices.

Serves 4

Total CHO   **60g**
Total calories 280

Orange Cool

25g/1 oz low fat spread
25g/1 oz fructose
2 size 3 eggs, separated
2 × 15ml spoons/2 tablespoons water
3 × 5ml spoons/3 teaspoons gelatine
225g/8 oz curd cheese

175ml/6 fl oz frozen concentrated
  orange juice, thawed

Decoration
thin orange slices

Put the spread, fructose and egg yolks in a bowl over a pan of boiling water and stir until the mixture thickens. Leave to cool. Put the water into a heatproof container, sprinkle in the gelatine and leave to soften. Stand the container in a pan of hot water and stir until the gelatine dissolves.

   Stir the curd cheese, orange juice and gelatine into the egg mixture. Whisk the egg whites until stiff and fold into the mixture. Pour into a serving dish and leave to set in a refrigerator. When set, decorate with thin slices of fresh orange.

Serves 4

Total CHO   **40g**
Total calories 820

Orange Jelly

2 × 15ml spoons/2 tablespoons water
3 × 5ml spoons/3 teaspoons gelatine
425ml/¾ pint unsweetened orange juice
1 × 15ml spoon/1 tablespoon lemon
 juice

liquid sweetener
orange food colouring

Decoration
thin orange slices

Put the water into a heatproof container, sprinkle in the
gelatine and leave to soften. Stand the container in a pan of
hot water and stir until the gelatine dissolves. Mix with the
remaining ingredients. Pour into a serving dish and leave to
set in a refrigerator. When set, decorate with thin slices of
fresh orange.

Serves 4

Total CHO   40g
Total calories   180

Rhubarb Snow

450g/1 lb rhubarb, trimmed and
 chopped
red food colouring
liquid sweetener
100g/4 oz cottage cheese

150g/5.3 oz natural yoghurt (1 small
 carton)
1 × 5ml spoon/1 teaspoon vanilla
 essence
1 egg white

Steam the rhubarb for about 20 minutes until tender. Add a
few drops of food colouring and liquid sweetener to taste.
Leave to cool completely. Mix together the cottage cheese,
yoghurt and vanilla essence. Whisk the egg white until stiff
and fold into the cheese and yoghurt mixture. Gently fold into
the rhubarb and leave to chill in a refrigerator.

Serves 4

Total CHO   10g
Total calories   220

Tropical Dessert

2 × 15ml spoons/2 tablespoons water
3 × 5ml spoons/3 teaspoons gelatine
2 small bananas

150ml/¼ pint skimmed milk
½ quantity of Mango Dressing (page 98)

Put the water in a heatproof container, sprinkle on the gelatine and leave to soften. Stand the container in a pan of hot water and stir until the gelatine dissolves. Leave to cool. Chop most of the bananas, and reserve a few slices for decoration. Mix the gelatine with the milk, bananas and mango dressing. Pour into four small glass dishes and leave to set in a refrigerator. Decorate with the reserved banana slices.

Serves 4

Total CHO   40g
Total calories 300

Natural Yoghurt

550ml/1 pint skimmed milk
1 × 15ml spoon/1 tablespoon natural
  yoghurt

Put the milk into a saucepan and heat to 43°C/110°F. (Use a thermometer to make sure that the temperature is correct.) Add the yoghurt and mix well. Pour into a clean vacuum flask. Close securely and leave undisturbed for 8-10 hours to allow the yoghurt to set.

   Store the yoghurt in a refrigerator. It will keep for up to 1 week.

Total CHO   30g
Total calories 200

Ices
Pineapple Sorbet

2 × 15ml spoons/2 tablespoons water
3 × 5ml spoons/3 teaspoons gelatine
1 × 225g/8 oz can pineapple in natural
  juice, chopped

3 × 15ml spoons/3 tablespoons fresh
  orange juice
ground ginger

Put the water into a heatproof container, sprinkle in the
gelatine and leave to soften. Stand the container in a pan of
hot water and stir until the gelatine dissolves. Add the gelatine
to the canned pineapple and juice and the orange juice.
Process in a blender, then pour into a 550ml/1 pint mould
and leave to set in a freezer. Serve sprinkled with ginger.

Serves 2

Total CHO   40g
Total calories   160

Yoghurt Orange Ice

150g/5.3 oz natural yoghurt (1 small
  carton)
200ml/7 fl oz unsweetened orange juice
  (1 small carton)

vanilla essence
orange food colouring

Decoration
fresh orange slices

Mix together the yoghurt, orange juice and a few drops of
vanilla essence and food colouring. Put into a suitable
container in a freezer and leave until partially frozen. Beat
well, then freeze until firm. Serve with slices of fresh orange.

Serves 2

Total CHO   30g
Total calories   160

Orange Sorbet

1 × 15ml spoon/1 tablespoon fructose
425ml/¾ pint boiling water
175ml/6 fl oz frozen concentrated
  orange juice, thawed

2 egg whites

Dissolve the fructose in the boiling water. Add the
concentrated orange juice, and mix well. Put in a suitable
container in a freezer and remove when on the point of
setting. Beat well. Whisk the egg whites until stiff and fold into
the iced mixture, then freeze until firm.

Serves 4

Total CHO   40g
Total calories   260

Pineapple Boats

1 medium pineapple
150g/5.3 oz natural yoghurt (1 small
  carton)

liquid sweetener

Cut the pineapple in half lengthways, scoop out and dice the flesh. Retaining a few pieces to use as decoration, put the pineapple in a suitable container in a freezer, and leave until almost frozen. Remove from the freezer and mix with the yoghurt and liquid sweetener. Use to fill the pineapple shells and decorate with the reserved pineapple pieces. Serve immediately. Each half is shared between two people.

Serves 4

Total CHO   **60g**
Total calories **280**

Strawberry Ice

3 × 15ml spoons/3 tablespoons water
3 × 5ml spoons/3 teaspoons gelatine
175g/6 oz strawberries, hulled

150g/5.3 oz natural yoghurt (1 small
  carton)
liquid sweetener

Put the water in a heatproof container, sprinkle in the gelatine and leave to soften. Stand the container in a pan of hot water and stir until the gelatine dissolves. Leave to cool, then add the strawberries, yoghurt and liquid sweetener. Sieve, or process in a blender. Pour into a suitable container and leave in a freezer until solid.

Serves 4

Total CHO   **20g**
Total calories **120**

Cheesecakes

Mandarin Cheesecake

25g/1 oz low fat spread
50g/2 oz wholewheat flakes (breakfast cereal)
2 × 15ml spoons/2 tablespoons water
3 × 5ml spoons/3 teaspoons gelatine
100g/4 oz curd cheese

1 × 225g/8 oz can mandarin oranges in natural juice
liquid sweetener

Decoration
orange segments

Melt the spread in a saucepan and stir in the wheat flake cereal. Press firmly on to the base of a 20cm/8 inch loose-bottomed cake tin and leave in a refrigerator to chill.

Put the water in a heatproof container, sprinkle in the gelatine and leave to soften. Stand the container in a pan of hot water and stir until the gelatine dissolves. Mix together with the curd cheese, mandarin oranges and liquid sweetener, and process in a blender. Pour on to the base and leave to set in a refrigerator. When set, decorate with a few orange segments.

Total CHO   *60g*
Total calories   *500*

Variation
Use pineapple instead of mandarin oranges, and make the base with 50g/2 oz margarine and 75g/3 oz cereal. Use only 50g/2 oz curd cheese. Decorate with a little chopped pineapple.

Total CHO   *80g*
Total calories   *680*

Blackcurrant Cheesecake

75g/3 oz low fat spread
175g/6 oz wholemeal breadcrumbs,
  toasted
liquid sweetener
2 × 15ml spoons/2 tablespoons water
3 × 5ml spoons/3 teaspoons gelatine

225g/8 oz blackcurrants
75g/3 oz curd cheese
75g/3 oz cottage cheese
5 × 15ml spoons/ 5 tablespoons
  skimmed milk
1 × 15ml spoon/1 tablespoon lemon
  juice

Melt the spread in a saucepan and stir in the toasted
breadcrumbs and liquid sweetener. Press firmly on to the
base of a 20cm/8 inch loose-bottomed cake tin and leave in
a refrigerator to chill.
   Put the water into a heatproof container, sprinkle in the
gelatine and leave to soften. Stand the container in a pan of
hot water and stir until the gelatine dissolves. Mix together
with the blackcurrants, cheeses, milk and lemon juice. Seive
or process in a blender until smooth. Pour on to the base and
leave in a refrigerator until set.

Total CHO   100g
Total calories 900

Coconut Cheesecake

75g/3 oz low fat spread
75g/3 oz wholewheat flakes (breakfast
  cereal)
6 digestive biscuits, crushed
2 size 3 eggs, separated

225g/8 oz cottage cheese
50g/2 oz desiccated coconut
1 × 15ml spoon/1 tablespoon skimmed
  milk
liquid sweetener

Melt the spread in a saucepan and stir in the cereal and
crushed biscuits. Press the mixture on to the base of a
20cm/8 inch loose-bottomed cake tin. Beat the egg yolks
together with the cottage cheese, coconut, milk and liquid
sweetener. Whisk the egg whites until stiff and fold into the
cheese mixture. Pour over the base and bake at
200°C/400°F/Gas 6 for 25 minutes, until set and golden-
brown. Serve hot or cold.

Total CHO   120g
Total calories 1440

Home Baking

Almond, Coffee and Apple Layer Cake

50g/2 oz wholemeal/wholewheat flour
1 × 5ml spoon/1 teaspoon baking
  powder
1 × 5ml spoon/1 teaspoon instant coffee
2 × 15ml spoons/2 tablespoons boiling
  water
3 size 3 eggs, separated
50g/2 oz fructose

2 × 15ml spoons/2 tablespoons ground
  almonds

Filling
2 large eating apples, peeled, cored and
  sliced
liquid sweetener

Sift together the flour and baking powder. Dissolve the
coffee in the water. Whisk the egg yolks and fructose until
thick and creamy. Fold in the coffee, flour and ground
almonds. Whisk the egg whites until stiff, and fold in carefully.
Turn into a 20cm/8 inch greased and lined sandwich tin, and
bake at 180°C/350°F/Gas 4 for 25-30 minutes.
   Meanwhile, steam the apples until soft, then mash them
and add the liquid sweetener. Leave to cool.
   Split the sponge in half and fill with the apple mixture.

Serves 8

Total CHO   60g
Total calories 860

Shirley's Anniversary Cake

4 eggs, separated
3 × 15ml spoons/3 tablespoons water
chocolate essence

75ml/⅛th pint skimmed milk
50g/2 oz fresh wholemeal breadcrumbs
25g/1 oz sultanas

Whisk the egg yolks with the water and chocolate essence
until fluffy. Add the milk, breadcrumbs and sultanas slowly,
mixing well. Beat the egg whites until very stiff and fold into
the mixture. Turn into a lined 15cm/6 inch cake tin and bake
at 140°C/275°F/Gas 1 for 1 hour.
   The cake can be split in half and filled with a little Slimmer's
Blackcurrant Jam (see page 134).

Total CHO   40g
Total calories 500

Slimmer's Blackcurrant Jam

450g/1 lb blackcurrants
150ml/¼ pint water

2 × 15ml spoons/2 tablespoons water
3 × 5ml spoons/3 teaspoons gelatine

Put the blackcurrants and 150ml/¼ pint water in a large saucepan. Heat to boiling point, reduce the heat, cover and simmer for 10 minutes. Put the 2 × 15ml spoons/ 2 tablespoons water in a heatproof container, sprinkle on the gelatine and leave to soften. Stand the container in a pan of hot water and stir until the gelatine dissolves. Stir the gelatine into the blackcurrants, and pour into sterilized screw-topped jars. Leave to cool, then store in a refrigerator.

Total CHO   30g
Total calories   120

Orange Rind Cake

50g/2 oz low fat spread
50g/2 oz fructose
2 size 3 eggs, well beaten
2 × 15ml spoons/2 tablespoons
  skimmed milk

100g/4 oz wholemeal/wholewheat flour
1 × 5ml spoon/1 teaspoon baking
  powder
grated rind of 2 oranges

Blend the spread and fructose until light and creamy. Gradually add the egg and milk, beating well after each addition. Fold in the flour, baking powder and orange rind. Turn into a 450g/1 lb well greased loaf tin and bake at 180°C/350°F/Gas 4 for about 30 minutes until golden and springy to the touch.

Total CHO   80g
Total calories   880

Raisin Wheat Bread

175g/6 oz self-raising
  wholemeal/wholewheat flour
1 × 5ml spoon/1 teaspoon baking
  powder
50g/2 oz low fat spread
2 × 15ml spoons/2 tablespoons fructose

50g/2 oz wholewheat flakes (breakfast
  cereal)
50g/2 oz raisins
25g/1 oz currants
2 size 3 eggs, well beaten

Sift together the flour and baking powder, then rub in the
spread until the mixture resembles fine breadcrumbs. Add
the fructose, cereal, raisins and currants, mix together well
and bind with the beaten eggs. Put the mixture into a 450g/1 lb
greased loaf tin and bake at 180°C/350°F/Gas 4 for about
30 minutes. Leave to cool before slicing.

Total CHO   200g
Total calories 1350

Oatcakes

25g/1 oz low fat spread
250g/9 oz oatmeal
1/2 × 2.5ml spoon/1/4 teaspoon salt

1/2 × 2.5ml spoon/1/4 teaspoon baking
  powder

Mix the spread with a little boiling water. Add the remaining
ingredients and mix to form a soft dough. Roll out thinly and
cut into 12 portions. Put on to a baking sheet and bake at
190°C/375°F/Gas 5 for 25 minutes or until lightly coloured.

Total CHO   180g
Total calories 1080

Parmesan Wholemeal Scones

100g/4 oz wholemeal/wholewheat flour
2 × 5ml spoons/2 teaspoons baking
  powder
1 × 2.5ml spoon/½ teaspoon salt
freshly ground black pepper
1 × 5ml spoon/1 teaspoon English
  mustard powder
50g/2 oz low fat spread

25g/1 oz Edam cheese, grated
25g/1 oz Parmesan cheese, grated
150ml/¼ pint skimmed milk

Garnish
tomato wedges
sprigs of parsley

In a large bowl sift together the flour, baking powder, salt, pepper and mustard. Rub in the spread until the mixture resembles fine breadcrumbs, then add the cheeses and milk and mix to a soft dough. Roll out on a lightly floured surface and use a pastry cutter to make eight scones. Put on to a baking sheet and bake at 230°C/450°F/Gas 8 for about 20 minutes until golden-brown. Garnish with tomato wedges and sprigs of parsley.

Total CHO **80g**
Total calories **800**

Yoghurt Wheat Scones

100g/4 oz wholemeal/wholewheat flour
1 × 5ml spoon/1 teaspoon baking
  powder
25g/1 oz low fat spread

salt
150g/5.3 oz natural yoghurt (1 small
  carton)

Sift together the flour and baking powder in a large bowl. Rub in the spread until the mixture resembles fine breadcrumbs. Stir in the salt and yoghurt and mix to a soft dough. Roll out on a lightly floured surface and use a pastry cutter to make eight scones. Put on a baking sheet and bake at 190°C/375°F/Gas 5 for 20 minutes until golden-brown. Serve hot.

Total CHO **80g**
Total calories **480**

Drinks

Drinks before or between meals can be very satisfying and real morale boosters, and some of those which follow will even convince you that you are not following a diet.

Chilled Coffee Cup

275ml/½ pint skimmed milk
1 × 15ml spoon/1 tablespoon instant
  coffee

liquid sweetener
6 ice cubes, crushed
grated cinnamon

Heat the milk gently, add the coffee and leave to dissolve, then cool. Add the liquid sweetener and crushed ice cubes, and serve in glasses with a little cinnamon sprinkled on the top.

Serves 2

Total CHO   20g
Total calories 120

Citrus Cooler

1 large orange, divided into segments,
1 very large grapefruit, divided into
  segments
1 × 5ml spoon/1 teaspoon ground
  ginger

550ml/1 pint cold water
2 × 15ml spoons/2 tablespoons cider
  vinegar
liquid sweetener
8 ice cubes

Sieve the fruit or process in a blender. Mix together with the ginger, water, vinegar and sweetener, pour into a glass jug and add the ice cubes. Drink from tall glasses with a straw.

Serves 2
Total CHO   20g
Total calories   80

Crazy Cocktail

75ml/⅛ pint sugar-free/low calorie
  bitter lemon
75ml/⅛ pint sugar-free/low calorie
  orange
150ml/¼ pint sugar-free/low calorie dry
  ginger

2 drops rum essence
ice cubes

Garnish
2 lemon slices
ground ginger (optional)

Mix together the bitter lemon, orange and dry ginger with the
rum essence and ice cubes. Chill in a refrigerator, and serve
in glasses with a lemon slice in each. A little ground ginger
can also be sprinkled on the top.

Serves 2

Total CHO   **neg**
Total calories   **10**

Fluffy Chocolate Cup

425ml/¾ pint skimmed milk
4 drops chocolate essence
liquid sweetener

Heat the milk gently, then add the chocolate essence and the
liquid sweetener. Whisk until frothy and serve immediately.

Serves 2
Total CHO   **20g**
Total calories **120**

Iced Mint Tea

4 × 5ml spoons/4 teaspoons mint
  tea (4 sachets)
550ml/1 pint cold water
6 strawberries, hulled

liquid sweetener

Decoration
fresh mint leaves

Brew the mint tea using 550ml/1 pint water and leave to cool.
Remove the sachets, if used, and transfer the tea to a glass
jug. Add the strawberries and sweetener, and leave in a
refrigerator to chill. Serve decorated with mint leaves.

Serves 2

Total CHO   **neg**
Total calories   **10**

Lemon Cooler

6 ice cubes, crushed
275ml/$\frac{1}{2}$ pint sugar-free/low calorie
  bitter lemon
2 lemon slices

1 medium red-skinned apple, sliced

Decoration
sprigs of fresh basil

Mix the ice cubes with the bitter lemon drink, lemon slices
and apple. Pour into a glass jug and serve decorated with
sprigs of basil.

Serves 2
Total CHO   **10g**
Total calories   **40**

Orange and Grapefruit Cocktail

150ml/$\frac{1}{4}$ pint unsweetened orange juice
150ml/$\frac{1}{4}$ pint unsweetened grapefruit
  juice
juice of 1 lemon
2 × 15ml spoons/2 tablespoons sugar-
  free/low calorie orange
150ml/$\frac{1}{4}$ pint cold water

liquid sweetener
ice cubes (optional)

Decoration
sprigs of fresh mint
2 orange slices

Mix together the fruit juices, orange drink and water, and add
the liquid sweetener. Fill cocktail glasses with ice cubes, if
used, and pour in the juices. Decorate each glass with sprigs
of mint and a slice of orange.

Serves 2

Total CHO   **30g**
Total calories **100**

Orange Strawberry Delight

juice of 1 lemon
75ml/⅛ pint natural orange juice
6 strawberries, hulled
550ml/1 pint cold water
liquid sweetener

6 ice cubes

Decoration
lemon slices

Mix together the lemon juice, orange juice, strawberries, water and liquid sweetener. Sieve, or process in a blender, and pour into tall glasses with the ice cubes. Place a slice of lemon on the rim of each glass.

Serves 2

Total CHO   **10g**
Total calories   **40**

Slimmer's Fruit Punch

550ml/1 pint sugar-free/low calorie
  lemonade
2 lemon slices
2 orange slices
2 red-skinned apple slices
2 strawberries, hulled and sliced

4 cucumber slices
ice cubes

Decoration
sprigs of mint

Put the lemonade in a glass jug and add the fruit and cucumber slices. Chill in a refrigerator. Serve in glasses filled with ice cubes. Decorate with mint leaves.

Serves 2
Total CHO   **neg**
Total calories   **20**

Té

4 × 5ml spoons/4 teaspoons
  camomile tea (4 sachets)
550ml/1 pint boiling water

liquid sweetener
1 large orange, sliced

Brew the tea using 550ml/1 pint water and leave to cool.
Remove the sachets, if used, and add the sweetener and
slices of orange. Leave in a refrigerator for 24 hours. Serve
cold, or re-heat and serve hot.

Serves 2

Total CHO   **10g**
Total calories   **40**

Tomato Blast

425ml/¾ pint tomato juice
1 × 15ml spoon/1 tablespoon
  Worcestershire sauce

Mix together the tomato juice and Worcestershire sauce and
chill well before serving.

Serves 2
Total CHO   **20g**
Total calories   **100**

Food Values

The food values listed below feature ingredients used within the recipes in this book. If you wish to substitute an ingredient, choose one from the chart which contains the same carbohydrate and calorie content.

Food	Amount	Approximate Carbohydrate Content	Approximate Calorie Content
Almonds, shelled	25g/1 oz	neg	140
Apple, cooking (whole)	450g/1 lb	35	135
Apple, eating (whole)	450g/1 lb	40	160
Apple juice (unsweetened)	150ml/¼ pint	18	70
Apricots (canned in natural juice)	1 × 227g/8 oz can	25	100
Apricots (dried)	25g/1 oz	11	45
Apricots (fresh, whole)	450g/1 lb	28	125
Arrowroot	1 × 5ml spoon/1 teaspoon	5	20
Asparagus (fresh)	450g/1 lb	12	60
Asparagus tips (canned)	1 × 298g/10 oz can	5	45
Aubergine (whole)	450g/1 lb	11	50
Avocado pear (1 whole)	225g/8 oz	3	360
Bamboo shoots (canned)	1 × 285g/10 oz can	12	80
Banana (peeled)	50g/2 oz	10	40
Beans, adukie (dried)	25g/1 oz	10	60
Beans, broad (fresh or frozen)	25g/1 oz	2	15
Beans, butter (canned)	1 × 425g/15 oz can	50	280
Beans, green	25g/1 oz	neg	5
Beans, red kidney (canned)	1 × 227g/8 oz can	30	165
Beans, red kidney (dried)	25g/1 oz	11	70
Beansprouts	450g/1 lb	10	50
Beef, minced (lean, raw)	450g/1 lb	-	800
Beef, stewing (lean, raw)	450g/1 lb	-	675
Biscuits, digestive (1 large)	15g/½ oz	10	70
Blackberries/blackcurrants (fresh or frozen)	450g/1 lb	30	120
Bread, wholemeal	1 large thin slice	13-15	70
Breadcrumbs, wholemeal (fresh)	25g/1 oz	10	55
Broccoli (fresh or frozen)	450g/1 lb	10	70

Food	Amount	Approximate Carbohydrate Content	Approximate Calorie Content
Cabbage, red (raw)	450g/1 lb	15	90
Cabbage, white (raw)	450g/1 lb	15	100
Carrots (whole)	450g/1 lb	20	100
Cauliflower (whole)	450g/1 lb	5	40
Celery (raw)	450g/1 lb	5	25
Cheese, Cheddar	25g/1 oz	neg	100-120
Cheese, cottage	25g/1 oz	neg	25
Cheese, curd	25g/1 oz	neg	50
Cheese, Edam	25g/1 oz	neg	75
Cheese, Gouda	25g/1 oz	neg	75
Cheese, Gruyère	25g/1 oz	neg	100
Cheese, Mozzarella	25g/1 oz	neg	100
Cheese, Parmesan	25g/1 oz	neg	100
Cheese, quark	25g/1 oz	neg	25
Cheese, ricotta	25g/1 oz	neg	100
Chicken (cooked)	25g/1 oz	-	35
Chicken breast (raw)	450g/1 lb	-	540
Chicken leg (raw, whole)	1 × 225g/8 oz	-	200
Chick-peas (dried)	25g/1 oz	12	80
Chinese leaves	450g/1 lb	15	120
Cider (dry)	150ml/¼ pint	4	55
Coconut (desiccated)	25g/1 oz	neg	150
Cod fillet or steak (raw)	450g/1 lb	-	320
Cornflour	1 × 5ml spoon/1 teaspoon	5	20
Courgettes (whole)	450g/1 lb	15	100
Crabmeat (canned or frozen)	25g/1 oz	-	20
Cucumber (whole)	450g/1 lb	5	35
Currants	25g/1 oz	16	60
Custard powder	1 × 5ml spoon/1 teaspoon	5	20
Dates (pitted)	25g/1 oz	16	60
Egg (size 3)	1	-	80
Fennel (whole)	450g/1 lb	20	120
Flour (wholemeal/wholewheat)	25g/1 oz	16	80
Frankfurters (canned)	1 × 227g/8 oz can	15	550

Food	Amount	Approximate Carbohydrate Content	Approximate Calorie Content
Fructose (fruit sugar)	25g/1 oz	see Note	100
Gelatine	1 × 5ml spoon/1 teaspoon	neg	15
Grapefruit (whole, unpeeled)	1 very large/400g/14 oz	10	45
Grapes (whole)	450g/1 lb	65	260
Haddock (fillet, raw)	450g/1 lb	-	330
Hake (fillet, raw)	450g/1 lb	-	330
Halibut (fillet, raw)	450g/1 lb	-	420
Ham (lean, cooked)	25g/1 oz	-	35-40
Lamb (lean, raw)	450g/1 lb	-	730
Leeks (whole)	450g/1 lb	10	50
Lentils (raw)	25g/1 oz	14	80
Lettuce	1 large	neg	20
Liver, calf's	450g/1 lb	-	690
Liver, chicken	450g/1 lb	-	605
Liver, lamb's	450g/1 lb	-	800
Liver, pig's	450g/1 lb	-	690
Mackerel, smoked (fillets)	450g/1 lb	-	960
Mackerel, fresh (whole)	450g/1 lb	-	520
Mandarin oranges (canned in natural juice)	1 × 298g/10½ oz can	20	80
Mango (whole)	450g/1 lb	45	180
Margarine (low fat)	25g/1 oz	-	95
Marrow (whole)	450g/1 lb	8	40
Melon, cantaloupe (whole)	450g/1 lb	15	65
Melon, honeydew (whole)	450g/1 lb	13	55
Melon, water (whole)	450g/1 lb	12	50
Milk, skimmed (fresh)	550ml/1 pint	27-30	180
Mushrooms (raw)	225g/8 oz	-	35
Nuts, pecan (shelled)	25g/1 oz	4	195

NOTE   The carbohydrate content of fructose is usually ignored by diabetics. It is important, however, that the maximum amount taken in any one day for diabetics is not more than 25g/1 oz

Food	Amount	Approximate Carbohydrate Content	Approximate Calorie Content
Oatmeal	25g/1 oz	18	100
Oats, rolled	25g/1 oz	18	100
Oil, olive	1 × 15ml spoon/1 tablespoon	-	135
Oil, soya bean	1 × 15ml spoon/1 tablespoon	-	135
Oil, sunflower	1 × 15ml spoon/1 tablespoon	-	135
Oil, vegetable	1 × 15ml spoon/1 tablespoon	-	135
Olives, black (stoned)	25g/1 oz	-	25
Onion	450g/1 lb	23	100
Orange (whole)	1 large/150g/5 oz	10	40
Orange juice (concentrated, frozen)	1 × 180g/6¼ oz can	50	225
Pasta, wholewheat (raw)	25g/1 oz	17	80
Peaches (fresh whole)	1 large/125g/4½ oz	10	40
Pear (whole)	450g/1 lb	35	130
Peas (frozen cooked)	25g/1 oz	2	10
Peppers (whole)	450g/1 lb	8	60
Pineapple (canned in natural juice)	1 × 225g/8 oz can	35	130
Pineapple (fresh whole)	450g/1 lb	28	110
Pineapple juice (unsweetened)	150ml/¼ pint	18	75
Plaice, fillet (raw)	450g/1 lb	-	400
Plums, dessert (whole)	450g/1 lb	40	160
Pork cutlet (with bone)	450g/1 lb	-	1230
Pork fillet (raw)	450g/1 lb	-	660
Pork, minced (lean, raw)	450g/1 lb	-	660
Prawns (peeled)	25g/1 oz	-	30
Prunes (stoned)	25g/1 oz	10	40
Rabbit (raw)	450g/1 lb	-	560
Radishes	450g/1 lb	6	30
Raisins	25g/1 oz	16	60
Raspberries (raw)	450g/1 lb	25	110
Rhubarb (raw, prepared)	450g/1 lb	5	30
Rice, brown (raw)	25g/1 oz	20	95
Rice, brown flakes (raw)	25g/1 oz	18	90

Food	Amount	Approximate Carbohydrate Content	Approximate Calorie Content
Salmon (canned)	1 × 99g/3½ oz can	-	155
Sauerkraut (canned or frozen)	450g/1 lb	20	80
Sherry, dry	150ml/¼ pint	2	170
Shredded wheat	1	18	80
Shrimps (canned)	1 × 113g/4 oz can	-	70
Shrimps (peeled)	25g/1 oz	-	30
Sole, lemon (fillet)	450g/1 lb	-	360
Strawberries (raw)	450g/1 lb	27	115
Sultanas	25g/1 oz	16	60
Sunflower seeds	25g/1 oz	5	140
Sweetcorn (canned)	1 × 350g/12 oz can	60	280
Tofu (soya bean curd)	227g/8 oz pack	7	115
Tomatoes (canned)	1 × 400g/14 oz can	10	50
Tomatoes (fresh)	450g/1 lb	12	60
Tomato juice (unsweetened)	150ml/¼ pint	5	25
Tomato purée	25g/1 oz	3	20
Tongue, ox (cooked)	25g/1 oz	-	60
Trout (whole)	450g/1 lb	-	220
Tuna (canned in brine)	1 × 200g/7 oz can	-	220
Turkey (fresh or frozen, meat only)	450g/1 lb	-	480
Veal escalope	450g/1 lb	-	490
Veal cutlet	1 medium 225g/8 oz	-	200
Veal fillet	450g/1 lb	-	490
Walnuts (shelled)	25g/1 oz	1½	130
Water chestnuts (canned)	1 × 284g/10 oz can	30	110
Watercress	25g/1 oz	neg	4
Wholewheat flake breakfast cereal	25g/1 oz	17	85
Wine, dry	150ml/¼ pint	1	100
Yoghurt, natural (low fat)	1 small carton/150g/5.3 oz	10	80

Index